ENGINEERING THE NEXT REVOLUTION
IN NEUROSCIENCE

ENGINEERING THE NEXT REVOLUTION IN NEUROSCIENCE

The New Science of Experiment Planning

Alcino J. Silva

Anthony Landreth

John Bickle

OXFORD
UNIVERSITY PRESS

OXFORD
UNIVERSITY PRESS

Oxford University Press is a department of the University of Oxford.
It furthers the University's objective of excellence in research, scholarship,
and education by publishing worldwide.

Oxford   New York

Auckland   Cape Town   Dar es Salaam   Hong Kong   Karachi
Kuala Lumpur   Madrid   Melbourne   Mexico City   Nairobi
New Delhi   Shanghai   Taipei   Toronto

With offices in

Argentina   Austria   Brazil   Chile   Czech Republic   France   Greece
Guatemala   Hungary   Italy   Japan   Poland   Portugal   Singapore
South Korea   Switzerland   Thailand   Turkey   Ukraine   Vietnam

Oxford is a registered trademark of Oxford University Press in the UK
and certain other countries.

Published in the United States of America by
Oxford University Press
198 Madison Avenue, New York, NY 10016

Library of Congress Cataloging-in-Publication Data
Silva, Alcino Jose Roriz Teixeira da, 1961–
Engineering the next revolution in neuroscience : the new science of experiment planning /
Alcino J. Silva, Anthony Landreth, John Bickle.
pages cm
Includes bibliographical references and index.
ISBN 978–0–19–973175–6 (alk. paper) — ISBN 978–0–19–932904–5 —
ISBN 978–0–19–932905–2   1. Neurosciences—Research.   2. Neurology—
Technological innovations.   I. Landreth, Anthony.   II. Bickle, John.   III. Title.
RC337.S55 2013
616.80072—dc23
2013005205

1 3 5 7 9 8 6 4 2
Printed in the United States of America
on acid-free paper

CONTENTS

ACKNOWLEDGMENTS

From Alcino J. Silva

I would like to recognize the invaluable contributions of several people without whom this book would have never been possible. First, my wife Tawnie Silva for her endless patience, for her wisdom and advice, for her love and selflessness, for being there when there was little else; my parents, and my children Alex and Elenna, for their unwavering support, encouragement, and many personal sacrifices that allowed me to work on this book when I should have been with them; my friend Alan Smith for nurturing the seeds that grew into some of the ideas described here; and the young scientists that worked in my laboratory over the years— their talent, imagination, and razor sharp intellects were the fertile ground in which this body of work developed. Finally, this book would have never happened without my co-authors; John Bickle for taking my naïve enthusiasm seriously, and especially Anthony W. Landreth for the intellectual courage to dedicate 3 years of his life to this project. His ideas, vision and clarity transformed almost every page of this book.

From Anthony Landreth

I would like to thank my wife, Kat Landreth, and my parents and grandparents, Christine and Mike Zimmerman and William and Shirley Clark, for their patience and support in the writing of this book. I would also like to thank the Carnegie Mellon Department of Philosophy for hosting me for a semester to learn the basics of graphical causal models. Special thanks go to Clark Glymour, Joe Ramsey, and Jim Bogen for conversations and lessons in the philosophy of science, and to George Graham for encouraging me to study philosophy of neuroscience in the first place. Thanks to the faculty at the University of Cincinnati's Philosophy and Sciences program. And, special thanks to John Bickle and Alcino Silva for the invitation to work on the project that yielded this book.

From John Bickle

I would like to thank my wife and lifetime partner, Marica Bernstein. Of all the things that life has thrown my way in a half-century on this planet, I'm most happy of all that the two of us are now living out our shared vision of joint human flourishing at our Farther Along Farm, amidst the red clay, rolling hills, and pine and hardwood forests of rural north central Mississippi. Thanks to three great step-daughters, Caroline Cooper, Kat Landreth, and Margaret Cooper, now all grown-up women, for enriching my life. Thanks to Mom and Dad, still going strong, in the closest life they'll ever get to "retirement." And many thanks, of course, to Alcino Silva and Tony Landreth, for putting up with my many worries about earlier accounts of these ideas. The initial ideas are Alcino's; the exceedingly hard work of putting them into initial written words was Tony's. My contributions were aimed at organization, presentation, idea development, and strength of arguments. This compelling project has now occupied us for more than a half-decade, ever since Alcino waxed philosophical one spring evening in 2005, sitting outside at the old Pavilion Restaurant atop Mt. Adams, overlooking downtown Cincinnati, the Ohio River, and the hills of northern Kentucky.

[1]

NAVIGATING NEUROSCIENCE

1. PLANNING EXPERIMENTS WITH A MAP AND COMPASS

Scientists often plan experiments using little more than their intuitions about what needs to be accomplished next. To the seasoned researcher, this procedure is akin to navigating a familiar but vast landscape without a map and compass. Scientists have been doing this for centuries now, since science's inception. This does not mean that experiments and research programs aren't often thoughtfully planned and executed. Scientists routinely think long and hard about which experiments to tackle next. But little prepares them to systematically scan the horizons of their field's potential. Good fortune and good mentors help some find successful routes among the many paths their research might take. Conversations with colleagues, journal clubs, and courses in experimental design offer some clues about how to steer research programs. But scientists won't find empirical research devoted to helping them decide how to structure a research program or what experiments to tackle next. In place of such research they will find only tradition, occasional lessons from their mentors, and their intuitions.

To extend our metaphor a bit: navigating over large, richly structured geographical areas without a map and compass is especially problematic. And hopefully it won't take much argument to show that even the current body of published neuroscience research—the terrain that experimenters must now navigate to review and plan experiments—is overwhelming. Over the past three decades neuroscientists have published more than 1.6 million articles, spanning increasingly specialized yet increasingly complex and interconnected fields and subfields. Already this is a corpus far beyond human reading capacity. This terrain of knowledge is rich and highly structured, but with our current resources we have barely tapped it. How many unrecognized but important conclusions lay buried within the vastness of this record? How often do we duplicate published work, or pursue dead-end experimental paths that could have been avoided had we been fully aware of the contents and implications of the full published experimental record, even in our own fields? How much published research has actually advanced our understanding of nervous system functions? What percentage of this published research instead represents little more than small variations on previous findings, retracing of familiar ground in the immense landscape of the published record? If we had a tool to help us both navigate the vastness of the published record and grasp its implications, how might this tool change the course of current and foreseeable research? Even the most optimistic principal investigator, grant reviewer, or journal referee has to admit that these questions lack easy answers. Yet we can no longer afford to continue to conduct research at current scales—and expense—without addressing them. The corpus of neuroscience research against which we now ask these questions will only continue to expand.

Our purpose with this book is to address those who see that there is a real need to change the way we navigate the published record and plan future experiments. Our most earnest hope is that this book will convince readers of the necessity and urgency to develop a science of experiment planning. The need for a systematic study of experiment planning is tightly connected with the urgent need for tools to navigate the immensity of the published record and inform experiment planning. Faced with increasingly complex research choices, neuroscientists now more than ever need new tools and new approaches to help guide their creativity and intuition.

2. A SCIENCE OF EXPERIMENT PLANNING

Statistics and the theory of experimental design enable us to answer formal questions about what can be inferred from our experimental data, given some assumptions about how the data were produced and how they are structured. But these disciplines operate at a level of abstraction far removed from many of the practical choices an experimenter must make when deciding how to produce that data. Experimentalists must either rely on existing paradigms or improvise when making these choices. There are no widely recognized principles to guide and inform experimenters' intuitions through the planning process, no systematic tools to help neuroscientists make these very important choices.

Before we go on and develop these themes, we will address a few questions that already may be troubling the reader. First, are we suggesting that we scientists don't plan our experiments thoughtfully? By no means. Do we doubt the power of scientific intuition? No, it would be silly to do so. Are we saying that we scientists possess no resources for systematically planning and evaluating experiments for relevance and importance? Again, by no means. Individual laboratories, grant review committees, journal referees, and research award committees think long and hard about whether a proposed experiment has promise for the field or about whether results from a performed experiment deserve publication. These processes of evaluation are hardly unstructured, arbitrary, or capricious. Many of the evaluative concepts scientists use to make these thoughtful and often difficult decisions will be ones we'll appeal to in this book. But what we are claiming to be missing is a unifying framework, a scheme that consolidates these evaluative concepts, an organized effort to systematically study and evaluate strategies we currently use to plan experiments.

In conducting experiments, neuroscientists ask and answer "first-order" questions about nervous system phenomena and their causal interconnections (see Fig. 1.1). Examples include questions about the relation of a specific kinase to learning, or the expression of a specific gene to memory retention. The ideas that we are interested in exploring here concern instead a different class of questions—questions about research mapping and planning. Consider a first-order question about a given protein's relation to learning. About that we might ask: Can we determine the weight of the evidence supporting a role for this protein in learning? Based on this evidence, what are the different ways we might study that protein's relation to learning? Given the experiments that have been performed on this relation and the results so far gathered, what is the most relevant experiment to try next? These questions are "second-order"; they are questions about scientific practice. We will therefore follow common practice and call systematic, data-driven studies investigating second-order questions about science "S2 studies."

To sharpen our statement of this book's guiding assumption: we propose that to answer S2 questions, we will need a framework of experimentation, a taxonomy, which will help us to organize both completed and planned experiments. Not only will we need

S2: a science that studies second-order questions.

Second-Order Question

What is the best way to study the relationship
between this kinase and learning?

.

.

.

First-Order Question

What is the relationship between this kinase and
learning?

Figure 1.1

a framework for the different kinds of information that different types of experiments can reveal, we will also need to be explicit about the rules used in combining the results from those experiments to infer neural mechanisms. We'll refer to this later process with the term "Integration"—that is, the process of combining results across distinct experiments. With a framework of experiments and the various methods of Integration stated clearly and explicitly, we propose to build maps of published research that will be used during experiment planning. The framework, the Integration principles, the maps of research findings we propose to derive from them, and their uses are at the heart of our discussion in this book.

We say that we will develop maps of research. This mapping metaphor suggests graphical or pictorial answers to S2 questions. Just as we might query a map about where we are geographically located relative to an unfamiliar landmark, so we might ask where specific lines of research fit among all of the other work that has been published on a particular scientific question. In later chapters of this book, we will consider how relying on a map of research findings makes it possible to determine where individual research efforts are positioned relative to other studies in a field. As the old saying goes, and every scientist knows first-hand, pictures often communicate more effectively than words alone.

Constructing a map requires a legend, a system with which to sort features of the landscape into meaningful categories. Any such legend will only be useful if it accurately maps the terrain. Map builders thus need field knowledge to ensure that they are charting the terrain accurately. In our case, this means expertise in the field of neuroscience we wish to map. We must be careful not to assume that the specific strategies used to build maps for one field will apply to other fields. And yet, we should not lose sight of features shared among fields.

For example, all experimentalists value *reproducibility* of results and *convergent* evidence. Different fields of neuroscience will pursue reproducibility and convergence using different instruments and approaches. For example, a cognitive neuroscientist will want to know how consistently the same behavioral protocol yields the same neural activation pattern in neuroimaging experiments (i.e., reproducibility). That same researcher may also want to know whether the results from such neuroimaging experiments agree with the predictions of a systems-level computational model (i.e., convergence). A neuroscientist working in molecular and cellular cognition, for example, may want to know whether a particular mutation in gene X reliably affects memory in the same way across labs (i.e., reproducibility). That same researcher may also want to know whether that gene X is activated during memory (i.e., convergence). Within their individual fields, these two neuroscientists both look for evidence of reproducibility and convergence.

That we can look abstractly at two very different experimental traditions and see commonalities in research aims should not be too big of a surprise. But not all research is experimental. Although reproducibility and convergence are just as important in computational neuroscience, the standards used to evaluate results in this field will include criteria that will look different from what we find in molecular and cellular cognition and cognitive neuroscience. Although computational models will often be held accountable to experimental data, and thereby inherit research strategies from experimental neuroscience, we should not confuse the project of mapping theories with the project of mapping experiments. Our focus in this book will be on mapping experimental research, because that is what is familiar to us. But, we should not forget the diversity of valuable research traditions outside of our framework.

3. GETTING CONCRETE

At an abstract level, all neuroscientists value reproducibility and convergence. But the strategies they use to pursue those value differ. We cannot be sure how well we are doing if we do not illustrate our approach with work from a specific area of research. How can we know whether our framework and principles will generalize if we cannot demonstrate that they apply to a single field?

So that we don't get lost in the clouds, we will illustrate our ideas as concretely as possible by discussing a number of case studies drawn from the published experimental record. To avoid errors of misinterpretation, we have kept the case studies discussed in this book within our scientific comfort zone. Our area of expertise is molecular and cellular studies of learning and memory. To put this point at the outset, with utmost clarity and explicitness: The system of experiment classification (i.e., the framework) and the methods of research Integration discussed here are derived from common implicit and explicit practices found in our subfield of neuroscience—molecular and cellular cognition (MCC for short).

The principles used in MCC reflect those used in other fields of biology where molecular and cellular approaches have had an impact, such as development, immunology, and cancer studies. We have not composed the framework or the principles we describe out of nothing. We simply made them explicit and propose to use them systematically for mapping and planning experiments in molecular and cellular cognition (Matynia et al., 2002). Thus before we delve further into the MCC framework and Integration principles, we will first introduce this relatively young neuroscience field.

The goal of MCC is to develop molecular and cellular explanations of cognitive phenomena. Neuroscientists working in MCC use a wide range of experimental tools, including molecular manipulations (e.g., gene targeting, viral vectors, pharmacology), cellular measures and manipulations (neuroanatomy, electrophysiology, optogenetics, cellular and circuit imaging), and a plethora of behavioral assays. The interdisciplinary experiments that characterize research in MCC reflect a large cross-section of approaches and techniques within current neuroscience. This makes our field an interesting place for the sort of S2 research we propose; potentially our S2 studies may be useful to experimenters beyond MCC. However, we expect that each major field in neuroscience—from molecular and cellular, to systems, to cognitive neuroscience—will need to develop their own strategies that reflect the implementation of fundamental research mapping principles such as reproducibility and convergence.

We will spend many pages of this book describing and illustrating our S2 ideas with specific experiments from MCC. Of course there are other experiments from MCC and from other fields of neuroscience that could be used as examples to illustrate our key concepts. We apologize in advance to our neuroscience colleagues for our admittedly biased illustrative choices. We simply used the examples we know best. We welcome descriptions of experimental practice and results from other fields that illustrate our concepts, and perhaps add to, refine, or even replace some of them. We emphasize that our discussions of MCC research are not intended as ends in themselves. Their purpose is to illustrate a system for mapping and planning neuroscience research. We hope this book will show that this general system is a tool that could be used by any experimenter in any scientific field.

Clarification of our purpose is crucial at the outset. A tool that some regard as an aid may be regarded by others as a hindrance. This is especially true when that tool is supposed to help experiment planning—an area of acknowledged scientific creativity and genius. Our recommendations for a science of experiment planning are no more intended to dictate the experiments a scientist *must* perform than an accurate map dictates a traveler's choice of future destinations. Our hope, rather, is that knowing with more clarity where we are, where we could go, and the ways we could get there, we will make better experimental choices as we move science ahead. As with any other tool, proven usefulness is the ultimate criterion for judging its worth.

4. BUT HOW MUCH OF THIS IS GOING TO BE NEW?

Before we even take our first substantive step, we recognize that some readers will be concerned or even apprehensive about our project. We've already noted that we'll be employing some familiar terms to denote key concepts in our framework and subsequent results—for example, S2 and Integration. Our concerns with the "pragmatic rationality" of experiment planning are shared by many philosophers and cognitive scientists of science, and those two groups haven't been bashful about offering and defending their recommendations. Even some rational decision theorists and economists have joined in this mix. Our map metaphor isn't novel. With all these familiar terms, concerns, and ideas, what exactly is going to be new in our approach and results?

No one should be surprised that many of our ideas will sound very familiar. How could this be otherwise? A lot of smart people have done some hard thinking about experimentation in science, and it would be completely implausible that most everything written prior to this book turned out to be misguided. It's equally implausible that three authors could construct an entirely new strategy for addressing questions about science, without employing a lot of work that has gone before. Of course we borrow ideas from others in what follows.

But there is novelty in these pages. Although the framework, Integration rules, and resulting research maps borrow terms and concepts freely from others, as far as we know the overall approach we propose is fundamentally new and its implications for neuroscience are far reaching. For example, the framework, Integration rules, and overall approach we introduce differs fundamentally from the "decompose functionally and localize neurally" strategy that has dominated much of cognitive neuroscience for nearly four decades (Posner and DiGirolamo, 2000). This point deserves a brief elaboration.

In the branches of neuroscience that have historically focused on explanations of behavior and cognition, the most popular experimental strategy has been first to understand the components and operations of the cognitive and behavioral function at issue (say, spatial memory) and then to identify the neural structures (e.g., the hippocampus, etc.) implementing the function's decomposed elements—hence the popular phrase, "decompose functionally and localize neurally." Neurocientists next investigate how these neural structures are connected to compose systems, then figure out the functional circuitries within each structure, and then unravel the cellular specificities of the circuitries and the intraneuronal molecular mechanisms that drive the cells' activities and dynamics. In other words, one could argue that the experimental project in much of cognitive neuroscience has been to work down a hierarchy of "levels," step-by-step, of both structure and function. The task at each level is to provide a mechanistic explanation of the activities measured at the next level up. Not only have many neuroscientists interested in cognitive and behavioral functions followed this strategy in their experimental undertakings, philosophers have speculated about the various ways that components and activities at each level relate to ones above and below (identity? composition? emergence? reduction? supervenience?).

No one should question the successes that this basic approach has achieved. Aspects of learning, memory, attention, motor control, cognitive planning, sensory experience in all modalities—you name the function—have all been fruitfully addressed by this hierarchical experimental strategy. Sometimes progress on a given function jumps around a bit across the various levels, not always following the idealized purely "top-down" path through the hierarchy sketched just above. But neuroscientific work on many cognitive and behavioral functions can be reconstructed without too much distortion of the actual history to reflect this experiment strategy.

Surely we're not advocating in this book throwing out this popular experimental strategy? Surely not. We fully acknowledge this methodology at work in neuroscience over the past four decades, the attempts to justify it philosophically, and the many beautiful scientific results it has engendered.

Yet, decomposition and localization should not be confused with the project of research mapping itself. Decomposition and localization are paradigm-specific values that also can be served by research maps. From a mapping perspective, we would like to find and map the experiments that support a particular decomposition or localization. To meet this kind of goal, we need additional concepts for classifying experiments and integrating their results. As we mentioned in the previous section, these additional concepts may sometimes differ in their details, depending on the research paradigm (e.g., cognitive neuroscience, systems neuroscience, MCC, etc.). It will be exceedingly interesting to compare useful frameworks and Integration rules across neuroscience fields, as well as their implications for experiment planning. This book's quixotic title reflects this hope: engineering the next revolution in neuroscience (not just in MCC!). We do not see this process as a single event emanating from a single field but as a multifaceted movement toward the development of a new science of research mapping and planning (S2). The multifaceted nature of this movement needs to reflect the diverse subject matter and research tools of each neuroscience field, without losing sight of the fundamental scientific values of reproducibility and convergence.

This discussion leads to an explanation of why MCC is an appropriate field for the goals of this book. In a nutshell, MCC experiments intervene into molecular pathways in neurons and attempt to develop explanations that bridge molecules, cells, circuits, and behavior. MCC has amassed an impressive experimental record over the past two decades. The corpus of results in MCC, like other subfields of neuroscience, has grown large enough to exceed its practitioners' ability to take it all in. Given the diversity of phenomena and techniques found in MCC—molecules and molecular methods, cells, circuits and physiological methods, behavior and behavioral methods—it is no wonder. If headway can be made in developing a strategy for mapping MCC, it should give us confidence that a similar strategy that includes a framework of experiments and Integration rules to combine these experiments should be possible for other fields. So, without further ado, let's start by taking a look at the framework we derived from MCC. After that we will introduce the Integration rules we propose to use in assembling research maps of MCC. This is a little book with big aspirations: we do believe that the approach described here could provide the tools and clarity needed for engineering the next revolution in neuroscience.

[2]

FRAMING MAPS OF RESEARCH FINDINGS

1. FIRST STEPS TOWARD A MAP

The maps in apps like Google Maps are drastic simplifications of the places they represent. The programmers and cartographers in charge of designing these maps needed to decide which entities to include (e.g., streets and landmarks) and which rules to use for accurately representing these entities (e.g. rules for scaling and color coding). These choices were made with the intent of helping people get to where they want to go. Too many details (or too many of the wrong details), and the maps would confuse their users. People would get lost. Similarly, in designing maps for neuroscience, we will need to make simplifying choices so that users can get what they want out of them. If a map app is there to answer users' questions about spatial relationships between locales, then a map of experimental neuroscience should answer users' questions about what is known, what is uncertain, and maybe even help them plan routes to future research.

In mapping neuroscience research we will need to decide how to organize the vast number of published experiments into a format that makes them accessible and interpretable. Organizing entities to be mapped (e.g., roads) into categories (e.g., surface streets, thoroughfares and highways) is a critical step in map design. Similarly, to represent experiments in neuroscience maps, it will be important to devise categories for classifying these experiments (i.e., a framework for classifying experiments). We will also need to come up with rules for how to integrate these experiments into a coherent map (rules of Integration). These rules should serve the evidential values of reproducibility and convergence shared among all neuroscientists. Let us consider the framework for classifying experiments first.

2. A FRAMEWORK FOR CLASSIFYING EXPERIMENTS IN MOLECULAR AND CELLULAR COGNITION

The neuroscience subfield we will focus on in this book is molecular and cellular cognition (MCC), a field of neuroscience that looks for connections among molecules, neurons, and behaviors associated with different forms of cognition (Matynia et al., 2002). Before going into great depth about research programs in MCC, we will present our framework for classifying MCC experiments in broad brushstrokes. In the next chapter, we will dig into MCC in greater detail, using case studies to illustrate the concepts in the framework.

Our framework sorts experiments in MCC according to their fundamental goals. As in perhaps other fields in neuroscience, one finds three basic kinds of experiments in MCC: (1) attempts to discover new phenomena and understand their properties (**Identity Experiments**); (2) tests of causal hypotheses (**Connection Experiments**); and (3) efforts to develop and characterize new tools for performing Identity and Connection experiments (**Tool Development Experiments**).[1] MCC is a field that has stressed connections between phenomena at different neuroscience levels, so far from molecular to cellular and behavioral mechanisms. The history of this field is marked by experiments connecting phenomena that were defined and discovered in other fields of neuroscience (e.g., molecular, cellular, systems, and behavioral neuroscience). Therefore, Connection Experiments will occupy much of our discussions. This is not to say that Identity and Tool experiments do not deserve the same or more attention: we had to start somewhere, and we have started with Connection experiments because they have had a key role in the field with which we are most familiar.

3. CONNECTION EXPERIMENTS

Most Connection Experiments in MCC involve manipulating a single variable (Single Connection Experiments) and measuring the changes on another. Occasionally Connection Experiments involve simultaneously manipulating two or more variables (Multi-Connection Experiments). Single Connection Experiments—testing some hypothesis such as A causes B $(A{\rightarrow}B)$—come in three different subvarieties. **Positive Manipulation** Experiments increase the probability of phenomenon A and measure for an effect on phenomenon B. For example, the use of a drug to increase the probability that a type of receptor (A) will be active in a specific brain region, and the use of a behavioral task to measure a specific type of memory phenomenon (B) known to be dependent on that brain region, would generally count as a Positive Manipulation experiment. The levels of the activity of A are increased, so A is positively manipulated.

Negative Manipulations decrease the probability of A and measure B. For example, to explore a possible causal connection between receptor A and memory phenomenon B, we could study the impact on B of a drug that blocks receptor A. It should be easy to see how the type of experiment described above (Positive Manipulation) compliments the experiment just described; the two use very different approaches to probe the hypothesized causal relation between A and B.

One problem with only using even clever combinations of Positive and Negative Manipulation experiments to test whether A affects B is that such experiments always artificially change A. Genes or drugs are used to increase, decrease, or change the activity of molecule A, thus altering pathways where these molecules function. Receptors and enzymes are inhibited or enhanced by synthetic pharmacological agents or by specific transgenic manipulations. Neurons are activated by embedded electrodes or by light-driven activation of artificial receptors (optogenetics). However, any changes observed in B may not necessarily result from a causal connection from A to B. They could instead be experimental side effects of the artificial way A was changed (manipulated). The experimental process manipulating A may also manipulate another phenomenon (C) in proximity of A. Although C is B's real cause, it appears to the experimenter, who is oblivious to C's involvement, that A instead causes B. This possibility reveals the need for Non-Intervention experiments to supplement Positive Manipulations and Negative Manipulations.

Non-Intervention Experiments measure A and B without manipulating either. These experiments help us to learn whether the relationship between A and B exists outside of an experimental setting. Without these experiments, it is more difficult to be confident that our other experimental results generalize beyond the artificial manipulations we designed. In MCC, convergent evidence among these three types of experiments (Positive and Negative Manipulations, Non-Interventions) is generally taken as good support for the hypothesis that A is part of the cause of B (*see* below).

As mentioned above, the categories of connection experiments reviewed apply to **Single Connection** experiments (i.e., experiments that test one causal connection at a time). However, there are MCC experiments that manipulate multiple phenomena simultaneously and look at the effects on another phenomenon. **Multi-Connection** experiments are simply composites of several simultaneous **Single-Connection** experiments. In general, Multi-Connection experiments help to unravel the mechanism of a single causal connection: How does A cause B? Is phenomenon C part of the mechanism by which A causes B ($A{\rightarrow}C{\rightarrow}B$)? Beyond testing the connection between C and B, to determine whether C is part of the mechanism by which A causes B, one would need to simultaneously manipulate A and C and then measure B (*see* below). If C mediates the effects of A on B ($A{\rightarrow}C{\rightarrow}B$), then Multi-Connection experiments should show that manipulations of C affect how changes in A impact B.

Since we've introduced a number of inter-related concepts quickly, it may be useful to illustrate them (see Fig. 2.1).

4. A STRATEGY TO ENCODE THE OUTCOME OF EXPERIMENTS

To assess the consistency and convergence of experimental results, we must attend not only to the manipulations and measurements performed but also the experimental outcomes. Therefore, experimental outcomes will be a critical component of maps of MCC. The outcomes of Connection Experiments can only vary in a few ways, and these possibilities can be used to categorize them: A change to the probability of A will either increase the probability of B, decrease

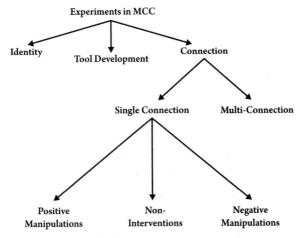

Figure 2.1 Components of a framework for classifying experiments in Molecular and Cellular Cognition (MCC).

the probability of B, or have no effect. When A's probability or magnitude is increased experimentally and B decreases, we have evidence for an inhibitory relationship between A and B. When A is increased and B increases, we have evidence for a facilitating relationship.

5. CONVERGENCE AND CONSISTENCY IN INTEGRATION

Consistency and convergence of results across experiments are the principal strategies used in MCC for determining the reliability of results, and the usefulness of hypotheses. Manipulations and measurements are used to generate data. Data are analyzed to make inferences about what happened in a particular experiment and how the outcome of that experiment comes to bear on the outcomes of other experiments. These inferences yield conclusions about experimental hypotheses—for example, that A reliably affects B or that A and B are independent of each other. Following the convention we introduced in the previous chapter, we'll refer to the process of analyzing the result of a collection of experiments as "**Integration**."

Two methods of Integration are directed at testing the robustness of a particular causal connection (i.e., **Convergent 3 Analysis** and **Consistency Analysis**, which takes the form of **Proxy Analysis** and **Replication Analysis**). Another method of Integration (i.e., **Eliminative Inference**) is used to assess competing hypotheses and eliminate alternative explanations for one experimental result when they conflict with the results of control experiments. The last method of Integration is directed at understanding how a particular connection works (i.e., **Mediation Analysis**). Together, the different forms of Integration help us to distinguish stronger hypotheses in the experimental literature from weaker hypotheses by uncovering patterns of consistency and convergence in evidence. (*See* Fig. 2.2.). Therefore, it is easy to see how these principles will be critical for assembling our MCC maps.

The names we have assigned to the different forms of Integration are supposed to be descriptive of the procedures they denote. Convergent 3 Analysis tests whether the outcomes of three different kinds of connection experiments (Positive Manipulations, Negative Manipulations, and Non-Interventions) are consistent with each other (i.e., whether they converge). For example, suppose we find that a drug blocks receptor A and causes a deficit in spatial learning. Suppose another drug that enhances the activity of receptor A also enhances the same form of learning. If we found that during spatial learning receptor A is activated, then our combined results would

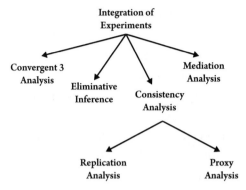

Figure 2.2 Components of the MCC Framework used to classify different kinds of analysis applied to collections of experiments.

make a compelling argument that activation of receptor A is part of a cause of spatial learning.

It is also important to assess whether similar experimental manipulations generally have the same kind of effect—that is, whether we have reproducibility of results. For example, we might ask whether different kinds of Positive Manipulations of a given type of receptor always result in an increase on a specific behavioral measure in a specific memory task. In looking for consistency among experimental results, we can demand more or less exactness. Proxy Analysis determines whether different but theoretically similar Connection Experiments have the same result. In Proxy Analysis, we can abstract from the details of phenomenon A, phenomenon B, or both A and B. For example, we can ask whether genetic and pharmacological negative manipulations of receptor A have the same impact on spatial learning. Replication Analysis, on the other hand, looks for consistency among experiments that employ exactly the same variables (e.g., the same receptor agonist, applied in the same way, with results gathered using the same task measures).

Knowing that A affects B is not the same thing as knowing *how A* affects B, or what is commonly referred to as the mechanism of A's effects on B. Understanding this mechanism increases our confidence in the causal connection between A and B. Generally, in MCC understanding the mechanism for the $A{\to}B$ causal connection involves the identification of mediators in that causal connection—that is, the go-betweens by which A is able to affect B. For example, suppose we know that spatial learning (B) depends on the function of some receptor (A). To understand how receptor A affects spatial learning B, we could start by asking what receptor A does that is required for spatial learning B. We might look for a protein (C) activated by receptor A that is also required for spatial learning B, such that $A{\to}C{\to}B$. We'll refer to this process of searching for the most likely mediators as Mediation Analysis, a process whose success depends heavily on Multi-Connection Experiments.

An example of a MCC Multi-Connection experiment would be to determine whether the enhancement of memory phenomenon B (e.g., spatial memory) caused by a Positive Manipulation of receptor A is affected by a Negative Manipulation of C. Showing that a Negative Manipulation of C prevents the enhancement in B brought about by A would suggest that C mediates the connection between A and B. Similarly, showing that the effects of a Negative Manipulation of A on B could be prevented by a Positive Manipulation of C (another example of a Multi-Connection experiment) would also be consistent with the idea that A causes B through C.

At the heart of most Integration methods is the familiar concept of evidential convergence—the notion that multiple, distinct lines of evidence are preferable to one line and that different types of experiments (Positive and Negative Manipulations, Non-Interventions) make unique contributions to testing the reliability of an hypothesized causal connection.

Beyond organizing experiments to be included in a map of MCC, the framework and Integration methods introduced here can also be used to find out what additional experiments could be done to further test any connection in a causal path. One of the key practical applications of our framework will be its use for organizing experimental evidence, and thereby revealing what we know, what we do not know, what we are uncertain about, and why, at any given time. Knowing what experimental evidence we are missing is helpful in determining which experiments to perform next. The more systematic and explicit we can render this knowledge, the more thorough the basis for these choices.

As we said earlier, the S2 Framework and Integration rules, presented in the diagrams and described so far, are derived from current research practices in MCC and in other fields that depend on molecular and cellular approaches (e.g., developmental biology, immunology, etc.). Yet key aspects of these will be familiar to most neuroscientists. We did not create the framework and Integration rules from first principles. Instead we lifted its components, piecemeal, from familiar concepts and forms of reasoning in MCC. Elaborating this S2 framework and rules and putting them to use systematically and explicitly toward mapping and planning experiments will occupy our discussion for most of this book.

6. MAPS OF EXPERIMENTS AND MAPS OF FINDINGS

In principle, it should be possible to take every research article in MCC, classify each reported experiment according to the framework introduced above, and build a database from a model of each experiment. All of the experiments that discovered the properties of every phenomenon studied in MCC (the field's Identity Experiments) and all of the experiments that assessed causal connections among these phenomena (the field's Connection Experiments) could be indexed to the Tool Development Experiments that made them possible. This database could then be graphed into a network where each node represents individual phenomena (defined by Identity Experiments) and the edges (i.e., links) denote Connection Experiments. It is also conceivable that such a network of experiments could be used to derive causal models (e.g., $A \rightarrow C \rightarrow B$), where each connection would be weighted according to its evidential strength along each Integration principle described above. Other things being equal, causal connections supported by Positive Manipulation, Negative Manipulation, and Non-Intervention Experiments carry more weight than those with support from only one or two of these (Convergent 3 Analysis). Similarly, connections with data that had been replicated independently are considered more reliable, and hence would receive a higher score in our envisioned networks, than those connections that had not (Replication Analysis).

We dream of engineering an interactive computer interface where one could click on any one tentative connection of this causal network and immediately be directed to the related published evidence. This computer system would be capable of taking the causal networks mentioned above and instantaneously highlighting the most likely causal path between any two phenomena of interest. Such a system would represent an enormous advance in our capacity to survey published experiments, and it would have myriad applications in experiment planning and evaluation. With such an interactive system neuroscientists could map previous findings and systematically and objectively evaluate specific research paths during experiment planning. They could share these evaluations and reasonably expect others in their field to be able to reconstruct the steps they took to reach that judgment. Imagining such a system, suggesting how it could be built, and understanding its implications for neuroscience are key goals of this book. But is any of this possible? Even if we had a scientifically justified S2 framework and Integration rules to accomplish this, do we have the technology to implement such a system?

7. THE IRRESISTIBLE DRAW OF THE SEEMINGLY IMPOSSIBLE

From a technological standpoint, the prospect of using a framework and Integration rules derived from MCC experiments to map research in this field may seem a distant dream. But it is not. Many of the requisite innovations have already been developed and are already used today for other purposes. We need only the proper intent to synthesize existing resources into tools fit for our purpose. In the later chapters of this book, we describe an approach to implementing the MCC framework and Integration methods using existing neuroinformatics resources.

Importantly, one need not wait for these technological innovations to start using the framework and Integration methods for experiment planning. As we'll demonstrate in Chapter 8, pencil and paper is all one needs to get surprisingly powerful results. Maps of specific MCC findings can be made right now! However, before we can draft any kind of map, handmade or otherwise, we need some grounding in real experimental case studies. Only by examining experimental results in some detail will we become familiar with the material our maps will need to represent.

[3]

A FRAMEWORK FOR MOLECULAR AND CELLULAR COGNITION

1. ORGANIZING THE WORLD WITH FRAMEWORKS

Organizing phenomena into categories (i.e., taxonomies) so that they can be more easily studied is important for all investigations. Physicists have categories of celestial bodies, chemists the periodic table, molecular biologists gene families, evolutionary biologists various phylogenies. Taxonomies enable us to catalog and organize the most fundamental information in a discipline, so that research can progress in an orderly and synergistic fashion. For example, by identifying a group of cells in a specific brain region as "glutamatergic neurons," neuroscientists reasonably assume that these neurons will share many of the properties common to glutamatergic neurons. Based on this classification, further characterization of those cells may involve a study of their action potentials, synaptic plasticity, and neuroconnectivity. If they had been identified as astrocytes, a type of glial cell, we would probably consider doing a different set of experiments.

A reasonable first step in systematically studying the principles behind experiment planning would be to catalog the different classes of experiments that could be planned (i.e., develop a taxonomy of experiments). In the previous chapter, we introduced such a taxonomy, the framework for experiments in MCC, and we discussed how this framework, together with a small number of Integration rules, could be used to map experiments in this field. In this chapter, we will illustrate the concepts of that framework more concretely with examples from hippocampal learning and memory studies. We will also provide a background in learning and memory the reader will need for the case studies we use in the rest of this book.

2. THREE FUNDAMENTAL CLASSES OF EXPERIMENT

Recall that at the root of our MCC framework, we listed three different types of experiment: Identity, Connection, and Tool Experiments. Experiments that specify the identifying properties of a phenomenon we call Identity Experiments. Identity experiments may proceed by describing a phenomenon's components, such as the various components of the hippocampal formation or the various regions of the hippocampus proper. (*See* Fig. 3.1).

The hippocampus proper consists of a pair of limbic structures tucked beneath the outer portions of temporal cortex, twins that curl onto themselves like sea horses reaching for their tails. Their name derives from "hippos" for horse and "campus" for sea creature. Although this structure was first named and described with Identity Experiments in the sixteenth century, it was not until the twentieth century that researchers used Connection Experiments to reveal its importance for learning and memory—specifically memory for events in one's life (episodic memory), for facts and meaning (semantic memory), and for spatial locations (spatial memory). The hippocampus proper is connected to other structures, such as the entorhinal cortex, that together compose the hippocampal formation. Inspired Identity Experiments by Santiago Ramón y Cajal at the turn of the last century revealed the morphology, neuroconnectivity, and other properties of the subregions of the hippocampus proper (Fig. 3.1). These properties identify these subregions as distinct from each other and other parts of the brain. As Identity Experiments articulate and refine our conception of a given phenomenon's properties and capacities (e.g., the CA1 hippocampal region), we also develop hypotheses of how that phenomenon affects other phenomena, such as memory. As neuroscientists describe new phenomena with Identity Experiments, conjectures invariably arise as to how the revealed properties of a phenomenon could be *causally connected* to changes in the properties of other phenomena.

Early neuroanatomical and neurophysiological studies of the hippocampus led naturally to speculation on its function. This in turn motivated studies that tested these ideas in detail. Many of these studies included Connection Experiments. In this class of experiment, we look for ways to manipulate the function of one phenomenon (e.g., lesions of the hippocampal formation) and then look at the impact on other phenomena (e.g., memory). We call these kinds of investigations Connection Experiments, because they are explicitly directed at probing and testing causal connections between phenomena. William Scoville and Brenda Milner's Connection Experiments confirmed previous suspicions that the hippocampus has a key role in memory (Scoville and Milner, 1957). Scoville resected the hippocampus of patient H.M. to treat

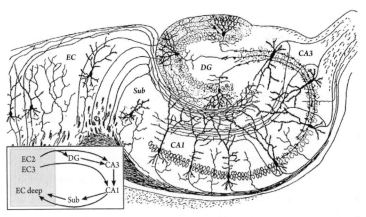

Figure 3.1 A sketch of the hippocampal formation by Santiago Ramon y Cajal, labeled with the contemporary taxonomy of hippocampal components. CA1 and CA3 are subfields of the hippocampus proper. Other structures of the hippocampal formation include the dentate gyrus (DG), the subiculum (Sub), and the entorhinal cortex (EC). Cells in different layers of the entorhinal cortex project to cells in different parts of the hippocampal formation. These components and projections were revealed by early Identity Experiments using neuronal staining techniques.

intractable epilepsy, and Milner characterized the surprisingly specific memory deficits that resulted from the operation: Most aspects of H.M.'s personality were untouched by the procedure, including his general intelligence, but H.M. had great difficulty in creating new episodic and semantic memories. Interestingly, he also almost entirely forgot events that took place around the time of the operation, although his older memories appeared to be spared! Scoville and Milner's spectacular findings motivated a large number of follow-up experiments that used a variety of techniques and approaches to probe the function of the hippocampus. In 2013, the Library of Medicine included more than 110,000 articles with references to the hippocampus!

To conduct Connection and Identity Experiments, we need instruments, tools that allow us to observe, manipulate, and measure accurately. This brings us to the third component of our taxonomy of experiments: Tool Development Experiments. This class of experiments includes those that are specially designed to develop new tools and to test their usefulness and limitations. Ramon y Cajal's classic Identity Experiments on hippocampal neuroanantomy took advantage of inspired Tool Development Experiments by his archrival Camillo Golgi. The Golgi stain that Ramon y Cajal used to generate his beautiful drawings of the hippocampus is a powerful neuroanatomical tool that continues to be used to this day. Similarly, Brenda Milner used a number of neuropsychological tools, including two tests developed by the American psychologist David Wechsler (e.g., the Wechsler-Bellevue Intelligence Scale and the Wechsler memory scales) to characterize the unexpectedly specific memory deficits of patient H.M.

The different kinds of experiment in our taxonomy specify an assortment of accomplishments that can be attained in neuroscience—knowledge of what a thing is (Identity Experiments), knowledge of what a thing does (Connection Experiments), and knowledge of how to measure and manipulate that thing (Tool Experiments). In the chapters to come, we will focus heavily on the accumulation of causal knowledge regarding MCC studies of mechanisms of learning and memory, our area of expertise. This will lead us to spend the preponderance of our discussion on Connection Experiments, the most developed thread in our Framework and at the very heart of the maps of MCC we discussed previously. Connection Experiments probe webs of causally linked phenomena that underlie maps of research. However before we can spin our molecular and cellular cognition web, before we can use the MCC framework and Integration rules to map research in this field, we need to introduce this area of neuroscience and trace back its historical origins.

3. CONNECTING SYNAPSES TO MEMORY

Scoville and Milner's spectacular results motivated a careful look into the mechanisms of hippocampal memory. Eventually, this led from lesion studies in animal models to physiological investigations and eventually to searches for the molecules involved in memory. The field of molecular and cellular cognition is a relative latecomer to studies of hippocampal memory. The field came of age in the early 1990s with Tool Development Experiments leading to techniques that allowed the molecular manipulation of any gene of interest in mice. Using these transgenic techniques, one of us (Silva) and colleagues in Susumu Tonegawa's laboratory (Silva et al., 1992a, 1992b) and Seth Grant and colleagues in Eric Kandel's laboratory (Grant et al., 1992) generated mice with mutations in genes involved in learning and memory processes. These and many other mutant mice that followed were easily shared among laboratories. The resulting multidisciplinary studies of these mice combined molecular, electrophysiological, and behavioral analyses and generated a large literature that explored causal connections between the complex molecular make up of the hippocampus and other memory structures, interesting cellular physiologies, and various forms of memory (hence the name, molecular and cellular cognition). Thousands of Connection Experiments carried out over the last three decades have demonstrated conclusively that a particular structure in neurons, the synapse, and its associated proteins plays a central role in learning and memory. But, we are getting ahead of ourselves. Before we delve into how synaptic proteins regulate the physiology of synapses and thereby affect learning and memory, we will first need to introduce the synapse and discuss some of the key physiological discoveries that motivated most of the work in molecular and cellular cognition.

A synapse is a structure that includes the presynaptic axonal terminal from which neurotransmitter is released and the opposing postsynaptic structure, called the spine, where neurotransmitters bind with receptors (Fig. 3.2) and trigger a complex cascade of signaling events that are central to learning and memory. Changes in the strength of synapses—their efficacy for passing charged ions selectively across the postsynaptic neuron—have long been suspected to be a mechanism for storing information during learning. This process of change in synapse strength is called synaptic plasticity. Early formulations of the synaptic theory of memory can be found as far back as the work of Alexander Bain (1873), but the most influential early account among neuroscientists was Donald Hebb's in his book, *The Organization of Behavior* (1949). Hebb wrote that during learning, "When the axon of cell A is near enough to excite a cell B and repeatedly or persistently takes part in firing it, some growth process or metabolic change takes place in one or both cells such that A's efficiency, as one of the cells firing B, is increased." In other words: Learning activates cells in relevant circuits and strengthens their connections. Over the 60-plus years that have followed, a huge number of Identity and Connection Experiments, investigating the properties and functions of hundreds of proteins, in multiple experimental organisms, and in several distinct brain regions have accumulated compelling, convergent evidence for the idea that increases in synaptic strength are a cellular mechanism for learning and memory.

A notable starting point for these experiments was work in Per Anderson's lab in Oslo, Norway in 1966. While working in

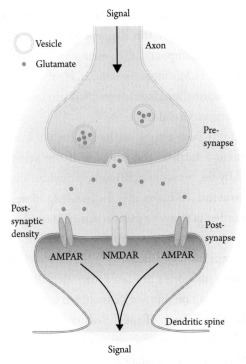

Figure 3.2 A chemical synapse consisting of the axon from a presynaptic neuron releasing the neurotransmitter glutamate into the synaptic cleft. The neurotransmitter molecules are transported intracellularly to the presynapse terminal in membrane-bound vesicles. On the opposite side is a segment of the postsynaptic neuron's dendrite (dendritic spine), where synaptic receptor proteins cluster (postsynaptic density). Here, the receptor proteins (e.g., AMPA receptors [AMPARs] and N-methyl-D-aspartate receptors [NMDARs]) regulate the flow of calcium and other ions that trigger a complex cascade of signaling events that have a role in learning and are critical for memory. Modified from Gécz (2010).

Anderson's lab, Terje Lømo found that he could detect stronger excitatory potentials from postsynaptic cells in the dentate gyrus if he first used high-frequency pulse trains to stimulate presynaptic cells in the entorhinal cortex (*see* Fig. 3.1). The preparatory train of stimuli, delivered through an electrode, appeared to alter the synaptic strength measured from dentate gyrus cells (Lømo, 1966; Lømo, 2003). Interestingly, this happened in the very structure of the brain (i.e., hippocampus) that Scoville and Milner had shown to be responsible for H.M.'s memory deficits. Hebb had predicted the existence of synaptic strengthening mechanisms in brain structures involved in memory. Could this be it?

After Timothy Bliss arrived in the lab, he and Lømo explored this phenomenon further, and found that the synaptic facilitation induced by the presynaptic stimulus could be measured from 30 minutes to at least 10 hours after the inducing stimulus, depending on the number of stimulus pulse trains (Bliss and Lømo, 1973). We now know that this increase in synaptic strength can last many days or even months (Abraham et al., 2002), which is important to note, because memories can last indefinitely. Bliss and Lømo's joint first publication on this work concluded with some hesitancy regarding the significance of their discovery. They were unsure of whether this facilitation and maintenance phenomenon could occur under natural circumstances. But the similarity that this phenomenon bore to some of Hebb's predictions did not elude them. They noted that the connection they found between the frequency of presynaptic signaling and synaptic facilitation could point to a physiological mechanism of memory formation. Due to the long-lasting character of this form of facilitation, measured, among other ways, as field excitatory postsynaptic potentials (fEP-SPs), this phenomenon was later dubbed "long-term potentiation" (LTP). Although our S2 Framework is focused on experimental neuroscience, these events show the importance of theoretical neuroscience work. Without Hebb's theoretical work, the potentiation discovered by Bliss and Lømo in the Anderson lab would probably have been regarded as little more than an electrophysiological curiosity.

Bliss and Lømo's discovery that LTP could be induced through the perforant path (i.e., entorhinal cortex to dentate gyrus) was followed by a flurry of other related findings that showed that it could also be induced in the Schaffer collateral pathway (i.e., CA3 to CA1; *see* Fig. 3.1) and in many other brain regions. Bliss and Lømo's pioneering Identity Experiments defined the fundamental properties of LTP and paved the way for a number of Connection Experiments to determine the relevance of this phenomenon to memory. Their results also raised questions about the mechanism of LTP itself.

Connection Experiments in the late 1970s and early 1980s suggested that increases in postsynaptic glutamate receptors are one of the causes of LTP, as the kind of repetitive stimulation of the hippocampus that triggers LTP also increases the abundance of postsynaptic glutamate receptors (*see* Fig. 3.2)(Baudry et al., 1980; Baudry and Lynch, 1981). By the time that these Connection Experiments were underway, numerous Identity Experiments showed that the amino acid glutamate was a prevalent excitatory neurotransmitter in mammalian central nervous systems. Thus, the greater numbers of these receptors at postsynaptic sites could help to explain the potentiation effects that follow the induction of LTP. Identity experiments showed that among the different kinds of glutamate receptors, some would preferentially bind an aspartate analog, *N*-methyl-D-aspartate (NMDA), and were hence called NMDA receptors (NMDARs).

4. THE AMAZING RECEPTOR

Identity and Connection Experiments quickly revealed that NMDARs have some interesting features. They can open to allow

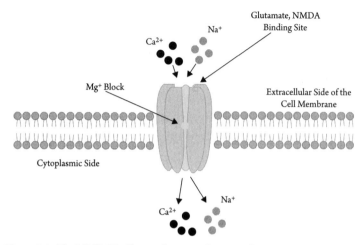

Figure 3.3 The NMDAR allows calcium to flow into the postsynaptic cell only under the conditions that the NMDAR has bound glutamate and the local membrane is already somewhat depolarized. When these two conditions are met, the magnesium block in the ion pore of the NMDAR is ejected, and calcium ions flow selectively into the postsynaptic cell.

calcium ions to flow across the postsynaptic neuron's membrane, but they will only do so if two conditions are met. First, glutamate must bind to the receptor, and second, the membrane nearby the bound NMDAR must already be sufficiently depolarized. When these two conditions hold, a magnesium ion blocking the NMDAR's ion channel is dislodged and calcium (and other ions) can enter the spine (*see* Fig. 3.3). Thus, the NMDAR appears to act as a coincidence detector for postsynaptic depolarization and presynaptic activity. And this is roughly what Hebb predicted three decades earlier—that is, that a synaptic learning mechanism would mediate synaptic strengthening through the simultaneous activation of pre- and postsynaptic cells.

In 1983, Graham Collingridge published a paper reporting Connection Experiments showing that NMDARs are critical for

LTP (Collingridge et al., 1983). To conduct these Connection Experiments, Collingridge used a tool to block these receptors' actions, a drug called (2R)-amino-5-phosphonovaleric acid (AP5, sometimes written APV). In that same paper, Collingridge also showed that blocking NMDARs did not disrupt normal cell firing in the hippocampus. These results suggested a provocative question: Could this new tool be used to block NMDARs during learning and therefore test the role of these receptors and LTP in memory?

It stood to reason that if LTP was part of the cellular mechanism for memory formation, AP5 might be just the tool to reveal this experimentally. Building on Collingridge's results in another lab, Richard Morris administered AP5 into certain regions of the hippocampus in rats (Morris et al., 1986). Morris then trained the rats in a task that now bears his name, the Morris water maze (Morris, 1981).

In the Morris water maze, rodents are placed in a round pool of opaque water, where they learn to navigate to an escape platform located in the pool. The platform lies just beneath the water's surface, hiding it from view. Once placed in the pool, the rat will swim through the murky water looking for any avenue of relief and eventually will escape to a point of rest when it finds the hidden platform. Placed back in the pool again, the rat will escape more quickly if it recalls the platform's location relative to visual cues posted outside of the pool. Otherwise, it will simply have to search the pool at random, all over again. (*See* Fig. 3.4.)

The rats that Morris treated with AP5 performed poorly on the hidden platform test—their time to find the hidden platform across numerous trials did not decrease nearly as rapidly as those rats treated with the control substance. But the AP5-treated rats did escape with normal latency when the platform's position was

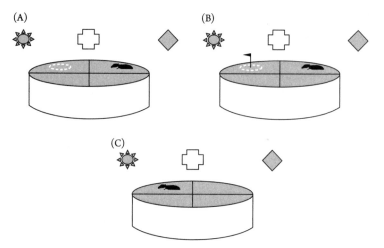

Figure 3.4 The Morris Water Maze with visual cues positioned around a room to enable a mouse or rat to orient itself in the water. (**A**) In training trials for the hidden platform task, the rodent is placed in the water at random locations and the escape platform is hidden just beneath the water's surface. Once the animal climbs onto the platform, it escapes the water and the experimenter removes it from the maze. Because the animal is released into the water from random locations during each training trial, it will only be able to learn which direction to swim if it orients itself using the room's visual cues. (**B**) In the visible platform task, a visual cue is placed on the platform so that the animal can see where the platform is located. The task does not depend on an intact hippocampus, but it does depend on intact visual perception and motivation. The visible platform is a control task for the hidden platform task. (**C**) In the probe phase of the hidden platform task, the platform is removed, and the experimenter records the amount of time the animal spends searching the quadrant where the platform was previously located. If an animal remembers the platform's location, then it will spend more time searching the respective quadrant.

visible, suggesting that their vision and motivation to escape were not negatively affected by AP5. Besides showing that they had a deficit in behavioral learning, Morris also tested his rats for LTP, in the same brain area where Bliss and Lømo had discovered it, the dentate gyrus. Consistent with Collingridge's findings, AP5-treated rats had a deficit in dentate gyrus LTP as well. All of this research suggested that rodent spatial learning depends on LTP and that LTP depends on the actions of NMDARs—a nice and tidy picture. Or so it seemed.

5. WHY WE NEED CONVERGENCE

A number of studies that followed, including Morris' own work, revealed that AP5 was having behavioral effects unrelated to learning (e.g., the treated rats seemed to often disregard the platform after stumbling onto it) (Cain et al., 1996). Further, careful studies carried out by Morris and colleagues showed that a dose of AP5 large enough to block nearly all dentate gyrus LTP did not seem to have much of an effect on spatial learning (Davis et al., 1992). These results were puzzling at the time, but as time went on, it became clear that disrupting NMDAR function in other hippocampal regions does affect spatial learning. But, the version of the water maze that Morris used is relatively insensitive to manipulations of NMDAR function in the dentate gyrus.

Addressing a hypothesis as complex and important as the role of LTP in learning would require 30 more years of experiments with nearly 200 other proteins, many of which are intracellular signaling proteins (e.g., kinases, phosphatases, and transcription factors) activated by NMDARs. Morris addressed the role of LTP in learning with experiments that impaired LTP (Negative Manipulation Experiments). Although powerful and useful, Negative Manipulation Experiments only tell us one part of this complex story. To convincingly implicate hippocampal LTP in learning, neuroscientists would need experiments that demonstrated that LTP does take place during learning (Non-Intervention Experiments)

(Moser et al., 1994) and experiments that showed that animals with enhanced hippocampal-dependent learning showed enhancements in LTP (Positive Manipulation Experiments) (Lee and Silva, 2009). The convergence between these three different types of experiments together with the sheer volume of these experiments demonstrating their robust reproducibility is what turned the corner in the LTP and learning saga. But new approaches were needed. Although powerful, pharmacology simply lacked the tools for this work.

The answer to this challenge changed neuroscience, and we will use the experiments that followed to illustrate the three different kinds of Connection Experiments in our framework. They provide three kinds of evidential thread, with each thread making a unique contribution to the articulation and experimental justification of a causal hypothesis. A framework allows us to classify experiments, but to use this framework for mapping previous results and planning future experiments, we need a set of principles, algorithms that capture how these categories of experiments could be used to both simplify the vastness of the published record and guide the process of determining which experiment to do next (Integration rules). Morris's seminal experiments were ground breaking but the findings were far from conclusive. This is not a problem of those carefully designed and very elegant experiments, but a characteristic of every single connection experiment. Any one experiment, no matter how influential and well designed, only tells one part of the story. The full account needs the convergence of complimentary experiments and the reproducibility of confirmatory work. Without the convergence and reproducibility captured in the Integration principles introduced in the previous chapter, we only have the promise of future discovery. The exciting thing about the framework and Integration rules mentioned is that they suggest very practical and straightforward strategies to analyze previous work and plan future experiments. These approaches are simple (they can be implemented with just pencil and paper), but they can have powerful applications.

[4]

THE POWER OF CONVERGENCE

1. NAVIGATING WITHOUT MAPS

Laboratory science is hardly roulette. But the process of planning and funding research does involve gambling to some extent. Funding agencies and donors bet on specific projects, and scientists use intuition and hunches to gamble their futures on a specific set of experiments. However thoughtful and careful these choices may be, with current tools critical data that could inform and instruct these important decisions may be overlooked because of the immensity of the published record.

Science and its products are part of the fabric of the modern world, but very little has been done to systematically study and optimize one of science's most critical steps: experiment planning. Research investments either pay off or they don't, and we take as normal and expected the fact that many, if not most, do not. Of course, the import of the information generated is not always immediate or immediately evident. Often it takes time for the value of the outcomes to be determined. Nevertheless, one would be hard pressed to find evidence that the majority of research publications in the Library of Medicine have had or will eventually have a significant impact. Undoubtedly, there are many reasons for this, but one of the reasons, in our view, is that we have been lacking the tools to efficiently and effectively explore, navigate, and interact with the published record. In other words, we lack research maps that could guide us through the sea of published material relevant to our work and to research planning. Without research maps, it is nearly impossible to track what has been done or fairly evaluate its significance, and without this information, it is increasingly difficult to place informed bets on future projects. Research maps will also allow us to track and study scientific progress in a discipline, such as MCC, and thus determine which approaches work well and which need improvement.

The payoff of a research investment is the provision of relevant and reliable knowledge, where a result is relevant only when it tells us either something that we didn't already know or confirms something worth knowing. Relevant results fill in gaps in our understanding, they allay our uncertainties when they converge with prior results, and occasionally they violate our expectations regarding hypotheses for which we have a prior interest. Where pieces do not fit, we will want to know why, and that too will help us to identify another source of research value.

In recognizing that there are different forms of research relevance, we must not slide into the mistaken belief that those forms are endless. The Integration rules introduced here summarize four distinct forms of relevance according to principles of consistency and convergence commonly used in neuroscience. Once we countenance the distinct ways that evidence can converge and be reproduced, we will be able to identify the kinds of research patterns that are worthy of completion. In other words, the Integration methods proposed are not only useful in evaluating the strength of evidence for particular findings, they are also useful for identifying research projects that are worthy of pursuit.

2. THE POWER OF CONVERGENCE

Each of the kinds of experiment in the MCC Framework (*see again* Fig. 1.1) addresses a fundamentally different question in science. Identity Experiments tell us about the defining characteristics of a phenomenon; they suggest how they may be potentially related to other phenomena, how to reliably identify the phenomenon by its measurable markings, and how to detect the phenomenon's presence or absence. In proposing the existence of a new phenomenon, we are betting on its demonstrable distinctness, on its importance within the network of other phenomena. Tool Development Experiments tell us that an instrument, or an approach, can be used to manipulate or measure a phenomenon with a significant degree of confidence. In this case, we are betting on the tool's accuracy and precision. Connection experiments tell us that there is a causal dependency, or independency, among phenomena of interest in a specific system. One common concern in Connection Experiments is that it is difficult to describe in detail how one phenomenon could cause another (e.g., How is it that the activation of NMDA receptors in the hippocampus is causally connected to spatial learning?). Not knowing *how* two phenomena are connected, we are left wondering whether the connection can really be trusted.

Another considerable problem is that the methods used to manipulate one phenomenon and measure changes in the other are almost always complex and poorly understood. For these and other reasons, there is always a real possibility that the results of any one Connection Experiment result from technical artifacts and from unintended changes in unrelated phenomena—every drug has off-target effects, every genetic manipulation has indirect effects on the expression of genes other than those targeted, every behavioral task is sensitive to changes in multiple brain systems. Were Morris's NMDAR results (Morris et al., 1986) a result of deficits in learning or in motivation or other behavioral phenomena needed for learning? It is difficult to be sure that the effects measured in any single connection experiment result from the intended manipulations. The key message in this chapter is that only the convergence of findings among very different experiments can give researchers the confidence that they are not being misled by their findings.

To elaborate our description of connection experiments, we will use case studies with which we are familiar. These experiments implicate calmodulin kinase II (CaMKII) in LTP and learning. Beyond our familiarity with these results, we chose them because they reflect an area of learning and memory research that captures many of the complexities of connection experiments in general. Before we start, it may be worth introducing CaMKII, our main character in the tale we are about to tell.

CaMKII is one of the most abundant proteins in synapses, and thus it is not surprising that it was one of the first synaptic proteins to be discovered (for a review of CaMKII's properties, see Wayman et al., 2008). CaMKII's name highlights a key aspect of its functional regulation, its dependency on calmodulin loaded with calcium for activation. Calmodulin is a promiscuous calcium carrier that, when loaded with calcium (e.g., resulting from NMDA receptor activation), changes its shape to activate a number of synaptic molecules, including the α-isoform of CaMKII (α-CaMKII).

Activated α-CaMKII phosphorylates other molecules. It picks up large phosphate groups from adenosine triphosphate (ATP) molecules and inserts them at specific sites on target molecules.

Recall that kinases in general—the "K" in CaMKII—are proteins that phosphorylate other molecules. Their activity is antagonized by phosphatases, like calcineurin, which remove phosphate groups from other molecules.

Phosphate groups change the structure and function of targeted proteins. Phosphorylation can activate proteins, whereas dephosphorylation can inactivate them. Many processes in cells are modulated by a carefully orchestrated tug of war between opposing kinases and phosphatases. For example, the elegant work of Isabelle Mansuy and colleagues has now shown that inhibiting certain phosphatases enhances LTP and memory, while increasing their activity levels has the opposite effect (Mansuy and Shenolikar, 2006).

3. A HOOK EXPERIMENT

When fields emerge and their research approaches are developed, there is almost always a novel idea, a powerful new tool, and an early experimental finding (a hook) to pique the scientific community's interest. In 1992, the field of Molecular and Cellular Cognition began with a series of such findings. Shortly after Morris's NMDAR findings, one of us (Silva) working in Susumu Tonegawa laboratory (Silva et al., 1992a and 1992b) took advantage of newly developed transgenic approaches, which allowed the mutation of any cloned gene, to test the connection among synaptic molecules, LTP, and memory. The gene chosen for these experiments coded for an abundant synaptic enzyme (α-CaMKII), which could be turned on by the activation of NMDARs. As we mentioned in the previous chapter, despite the impact of Morris's visionary and pioneering experiments with NMDAR blockers, there were concerns and ucertainties related to the non-learning effects of the drug used (AP5)

(Cain et al., 1996), and the finding that conditions that blocked nearly all dentate gyrus LTP did not seem to prevent learning (Davis et al., 1992). Unfortunately, at the time there were not many other drugs that could be used to test the tantalizing connection among NMDAR-dependent synaptic processes, LTP, and learning. Could novel transgenic methods provide a way to manipulate synaptic genes involved in LTP and therefore test the role of this fascinating phenomenon in memory?

Prior to transgenic experiments with α^-CaMKII in the early 1990s, modeling efforts had already suggested that a molecule with the properties of this kinase might be relevant for understanding how NMDARs affect synaptic plasticity and learning. The idea, first articulated by John Lisman, was fairly simple (Lisman, 1985, 1988). Start with a protein kinase, an enzyme that modulates other proteins by adding to them a phosphate group. Assume that when calcium flows into the postsynaptic membrane through NMDARs, this synaptic kinase goes into an active state. If that kinase can stay active after the calcium influx has subsided, and if by its activity it can strengthen synapses, then that kinase could act as a mechanism for holding on to memories, at least for a short time. So now neuroscience had Hebb's powerful general model for learning, and Lisman's more specific model for how information could be captured by molecules in real synapses and neurons.

In 1986, Stephen Miller and Mary Kennedy published a paper reporting elegant Identity Experiments, demonstrating that CaMKII had many of the biochemical properties that Lisman's model had predicted (Miller and Kennedy, 1986). However, to test Lisman's model, one would need to be able to manipulate CaMKII specifically in a living, behaving animal, and then test the impact of these manipulations (e.g., deletion of the kinase) on both synaptic function and behavior. This was a tall experimental order, in view of the tools available in the 1980s.

In science, however, one decade's impossible experiment is another decade's routine procedure. The 1992 α-CaMKII studies showed that this mutation disrupted hippocampal LTP and hippocampal learning (Silva et al., 1992a, 1992b). Lisman and Kennedy's work had suggested that deleting this hippocampal kinase should interfere with both hippocampal synaptic plasticity and learning tasks that depend on hippocampus function.

The α-CaMKII mice were engineered using gene-targeting techniques that had recently been developed (Silva et al., 1992a). In 2007 Mario R. Capecchi, Martin J. Evans, and Oliver Smithies won the Nobel Prize for their role in these Tool Development Experiments. With the techniques their laboratories developed, it became possible to alter or delete any cloned gene of interest (Capecchi, 1989). The gene is first mutated in embryonic stem cells, and then these cells are used to colonize host embryos, and eventually generate genetic lines of mice with the mutation in every cell (e.g., α-CaMKII mutant mice). Because α-CaMKII is almost exclusively expressed in post-natal forebrain excitatory neurons, the mutation did not compromise the survival or the general health of the mutant mice. After confirming that the mutation eliminated α-CaMKII without affecting other closely related kinases, the mice were used in hippocampal LTP studies. Electrophysiological studies (with Yan-Yan Wang in Chuck Stevens laboratory) revealed that the α-CaMKII deletion caused clear deficits in LTP measured in the CA1 region of the hippocampus, a region critical for the learning tasks used to test the mice (Silva et al., 1992a). Behavioral studies (with Richard Paylor in Jeanne Wehner's laboratory) showed that the α-CaMKII mutant mice had severe deficits in multiple hippocampal learning tests (Silva et al., 1992b). For example, the mutants took many more trials than their normal siblings to learn the location of the hidden platform in Morris's water maze.

The α-CaMKII knockouts were also tested in contextual fear conditioning, another test sensitive to changes in hippocampal function. In this test, a mouse is placed in a chamber with a grid floor, and after a couple of minutes of free exploratory time, it receives a mild foot shock through the grid. The pairing of the novel context (chamber) with the mild shock drives the mouse to associate the two, and therefore to fear the chamber. Freezing—a state of motionlessness—is one of the ways mice express fear behaviorally. (*See* Fig. 4.1.) Altogether the water maze and fear conditioning results suggested that the α-CaMKII mutation disrupted hippocampal learning, because the mutant mice not only showed spatial learning deficits, they also failed to exhibited little to no freezing when retested in the training context. Lisman's and Hebb's ideas appeared to have real experimental merit!

Soon after the α-CaMKII papers came out, Seth Grant, Tom O'Dell and colleagues in Eric Kandel's laboratory reported studies with mice with knockout mutations of the Fyn Tyrosine kinase previously derived for cancer studies in Phil Soriano's laboratory. Grant and O'Dell showed that the Fyn knockouts had deficient CA1 LTP and learning impairments in the Morris water maze and contextual fear conditioning (Grant et al., 1992). The convergence among the α-CaMKII, Fyn genetic findings, and Morris' AP5 experiments was striking. In all three cases, manipulations that blocked hippocampal LTP also blocked hippocampal learning.

These early transgenic studies integrating biochemistry, physiology, and behavior attracted a considerable amount of attention because of the potential promise of this experimental approach for studies of behavioral mechanisms. But honeymoons are invariably short in science, as initial enthusiasm and excitement with new

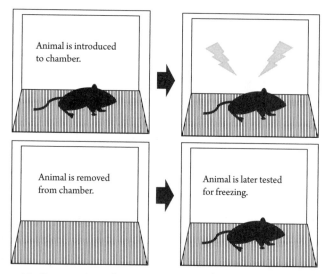

Figure 4.1 Contextual conditioning. An animal (e.g., a mouse) is placed in a conditioning chamber and allowed to explore the environment. Then, after a couple of minutes when the mouse has an opportunity to get acquainted with the chamber, a mild shock is delivered through the grid of the chamber to the animal's feet. This mild shock teaches the animal to fear this environment. The animal is removed from the chamber and then later placed back in the conditioning chamber. The animal expresses its memory of the chamber by freezing—that is, an evolutionarily adaptive reaction to fear because most predators are very good at detecting motion.

discoveries is quickly replaced by healthy skepticism and close scrutiny over the power and limitations of the new experimental tools.

4. UNCERTAINTY AND CONVERGENCE IN SCIENCE

The initial knockout experiments with α-CaMKII and Fyn raised important questions. How could manipulating proteins expressed throughout much of the forebrain affect hippocampal-dependent learning specifically? Both kinases are expressed in post-natal development, and therefore the learning deficits of the mutant mice could conceivably be unrelated to their deficits in LTP and rather result from faulty hippocampal development. Consistent with this view, the Fyn kinase mutation caused visible alterations in hippocampal structure. Could these structural changes, and not the abnormalities in LTP, be responsible for the learning deficits of the Fyn knockouts? Were these experiments the beginning of a new paradigm or merely a novelty? Could the general approach introduced in these publications be used to unravel mechanisms of behavior, or were there fundamental problems and confounds that would make this approach limited, or even useless? These questions draw our attention to the most central and pressing questions of S2, questions whose answers rely ultimately on convergent and reproducible evidence. How can we know when the results of experiments are robust and reliable? How can we distinguish between a productive paradigm and a flashy but ultimately sterile new approach? And how can we justify any answers we give to these questions in a responsible, systematic manner?

5. WHEN IT'S MUTUAL: CONVERGENT
3 ANALYSES

If we can trust the experimental evidence suggesting that CaMKII activation affects LTP, then we can rely on this hypothesis to study phenomena mediating CaMKII activation and synaptic potentiation. If we can trust the evidence that LTP affects learning, then we can look for mediators there as well. But if these hypotheses were untrustworthy, if we had evidence contrary to the results of these experiments, then we would be unadvised to build larger hypotheses out of them.

How can we assess the dependability of the proposed connection between CaMKII activation and LTP? For the sake of brevity and simplicity, the hypothetical link between two phenomena, such as CaMKII and LTP, is often represented with an arrow (CaMKII → LTP), a deceptively innocent-looking symbol. What the arrow represents is that the probability of LTP occurring depends on the probability of some activity of CaMKII. Setting technical limitations aside, molecular and cellular neuroscientists usually carry out at least three fundamentally different types of experiments to test connections such as "CaMKII activation→LTP":

1. They study CaMKII activation during LTP without manipulating CaMKII or LTP.
2. They decrease the levels or activity of CaMKII and measure the impact on LTP.
3. They increase the levels of CaMKII and again measure the impact on LTP.

If the results of these three types of experiments are consistent (i.e., convergent) and the results can be reproduced, they then support the hypothesis that CaMKII is a contributing cause (but not necessarily *the only* cause!) of LTP.

Initially the "CaMKII → LTP" hypothesis was tested with multiple pharmacological and genetic manipulations that decreased CaMKII levels in rats and mice, and in all cases there was a loss of hippocampal CA1 LTP. Despite the differences in manipulations used, these experiments are mutually relevant to testing the causal hypothesis, CaMKII activation→LTP. They all test the same hypothesis. Now suppose that all experiments confirm the dependency, CaMKII→LTP, and that their results are consistent with the other two types of experiments (i.e., those that increase the levels of CaMKII activation and enhance LTP, and those that observe CaMKII activation during LTP induction). In that happy case, all results converge. If we detect their convergence, then we have *integrated* these results into a case for the causal hypothesis, CaMKII activation→LTP.

How many basic kinds of Connection Experiments can converge on the same causal hypothesis? As previously outlined, we propose that there are at least three fundamentally different general classes of Connection Experiments. One type of Connection Experiment (Non-Intervention) involves no direct experimental manipulation of the hypothesized causal agent—in this case, CaMKII. For example, finding that CaMKII is activated during LTP induction would not demonstrate either that the kinase is needed or even causally involved in LTP, but it is consistent with the idea that the kinase *could be* involved in LTP. On the other hand, failing to find any change in the functional state of CaMKII during LTP induction would be inconsistent with the causal hypothesis, CaMKII activation→LTP. From measurements of CaMKII activation and LTP, we can estimate the probability that there will be LTP following activation of CaMKII. Assuming that we have the tools to measure these two events separately in the same experiment, and that we have the required time resolution, we can investigate whether increases in CaMKII activation precede the increases in synaptic strength that characterize LTP. Because these measurements of CaMKII and LTP do not involve deliberate experimental interventions on the agent (i.e., CaMKII) or target (i.e., LTP) we call these Non-Intervention Experiments. Of course, for such experiments to be conducted, a skull will have to be opened and measurements taken in the brain or in brain slices. These manipulations are hardly

"Non-Interventions." However, they are designed not to manipulate the variables of interest but, rather, to set up conditions for the required observations. Because most experiments have unintended consequences, it is important to show through control experiments that there is no reason to attribute the results of Non-Interventions to such incidental effects. We will discuss control experiments in more depth later on.

If Non-Intervention Experiments reveal that the states of a hypothesized causal agent (e.g., CaMKII) and (one of its) target effects (e.g., LTP) are reasonably correlated (when one goes up the other follows, etc.), we may still wonder whether the agent's state is responsible for the target's state. For example, there might be a common cause for both phenomena, one of the reasons why Non-Intervention results alone are not sufficient to establish a causal connection. But if we can manipulate the hypothesized causal agent directly, it will be much easier for us to determine whether the "agent" A is driving the effect B of interest or if some other phenomenon C is independently driving the two $(A \leftarrow C \rightarrow B)$. If A causes B, then manipulating A will affect B. If A and B are correlated solely because they share common cause C, then manipulating A might not affect B.

When neuroscientists manipulate a hypothesized causal agent, there are only two probabilistic directions for the manipulation to move. Either we *reduce* the probability that the agent will assume some state or we *increase* it. When we increase the probability of the agent assuming some state, we have performed a *Positive Manipulation*, and when we decrease it, we have performed a *Negative Manipulation*.

If neuroscientists decrease the levels of CaMKII available in a synapse—for example, by deleting the gene that codes for one of the isoforms of this kinase—then they will have performed a

Negative Manipulation.[1] If they increase the levels of CaMKII in the synapse—for example, with a transgenic manipulation that over expresses the kinase—then they will have performed a Positive Manipulation. One experiment reduces the probability of available activated CaMKII, whereas the other increases that probability (*see* Fig. 2.1).

These three different kinds of Connection Experiment— Positive and Negative Manipulations and Non-Interventions— each produce distinct kinds of evidence for a hypothesized causal dependency. And each kind has its own limitations. A Negative Manipulation, for example, can reveal that A is necessary for B to occur.[2] But that same Negative Manipulation cannot show that A normally causes B, nor can it distinguish between *triggering causes* of B and *background conditions* for B (*see* below). This has important consequences for experimental evidence.

If we were to cut the blood supply to an animal's hippocampus, then we would quickly and dramatically change synaptic plasticity, including LTP in the CA1 region. However, this result wouldn't show us that hippocampal blood supply normally causes LTP in these cells. Rather, we would get this result because the procedure unleashed a cascade of events that dramatically changed the general health and function of CA1 cells. A constant supply of blood to the hippocampus is a *background condition* for the normal regulation of synaptic plasticity, including LTP in CA1 cells. Thus, a Negative Manipulation alone cannot demonstrate whether one phenomenon is the *triggering cause* of another.

Under certain conditions, a Positive Manipulation can show us that A is part of a sufficient condition for triggering B. But again, a Positive Manipulation alone cannot show that A is a normal cause of B. For example, Guosong Liu and colleagues demonstrated that increasing the levels of brain magnesium in laboratory rats can result in enhancements in hippocampal-dependent learning. However, the authors did not conclude that magnesium triggers hippocampal learning (e.g., there are no known increases in the levels of magnesium during learning). Rather, proper levels of magnesium and an appropriate blood supply are considered background conditions for learning. Li's work simply suggests that modern diets are unfortunately impoverished in magnesium (Slutsky et al., 2010).

Non-Intervention Experiments can show that A's occurrences normally are correlated with B's and, in cases where the experiment has the appropriate temporal resolution, might also show that A occurs before B. As we stated before, Non-Intervention Experiments alone do not show that A causes B. We are reminded of the popular dictum that correlation does equal causation. We would like to propose extending the meaning of this dictum to Positive and Negative Manipulation Experiments. To generate compelling evidence for causation, we need to *integrate* across the results of these three different kinds of Connection Experiments. Convergent results with these three very different types of experiments help to make a compelling case that A is part of the cause of B (again, we would still need to show that each of these results is reproducible). Arthur Conan Doyle said it best through his character Sherlock Holmes: "We must look for consistency. Where there is a want of it we must suspect deception."

It is important to note that what Positive and Negative Manipulations reveal depends on the configuration of the causal system being investigated. An analogy might be helpful. Consider two homes, one with a well-fueled back-up generator (a redundant system) and one without. In both cases, the utility lines normally power these homes, but when the utility line to one of them is cut, the back-up generator will kick in. Cutting the utility line (Negative Manipulation) of the house with the redundant system would not affect the availability of power. However, on the non-redundant system, the Negative Manipulation would interrupt power to the house, showing the importance of the utility line. This analogy illustrates the need for convergent evidence. Without additional information, the Negative Manipulation described above would suggest that the utility line was not causally related to the power supply for the house.

We could use the same analogy to illustrate how the configuration of the causal system could affect the results of Positive Manipulations. Imagine that to determine the function of the generator we decide to add another one to the system. If the existing power supply is sufficient for the energy requirements of the house, then we may not be able to see the benefits of adding a second generator. However, if the power supplied to the house were insufficient, then one would see the benefits of adding an additional generator. The lack of an expected result with either a Positive or Negative Manipulation is not sufficient to discount a given hypothesis. No matter how well designed, single experiments can only tell us part of the story. This applies to the process of either supporting or refuting a hypothesis. If the whole story is what we are looking for, then there is no way around convergence.

6. THE EYE ON THE TARGET

So far in our examples of Connection Experiments, we focused our attention on facilitating causal connections (increases in the Agent lead to increases in the Target). However, there are a number of other types of Positive and Negative Manipulations that can be differentiated by focusing on the effects on the Target (*see* Fig. 4.2), and they too make unique contributions to the evaluation of causal

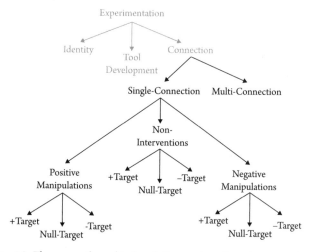

Figure 4.2 There are three kinds of Connection Experiment within the S2 Framework and three different subtypes of each kind of Connection Experiment. Positive Manipulations increase the probability of the Agent. Negative Manipulations decrease the probability of the Agent. Non-Interventions measure the Agent and Target without tampering with the Agent. Target-Increase Experiments result in an increase in the probability of the Target. Target-Decrease Experiments result in a decrease in the probability of the Target. Null-Target Experiments show that the Agent does not affect the Target in a particular experimental context. Non-Intervention Experiments measure correlation without manipulations, so the outcomes are either Positive Correlation (more A leads to more B or less A leads to less B), Negative Correlation (more A leads to less B or less A leads to more B), and Null Correlation (A and B are uncorrelated).

hypotheses. For example, Negative Manipulations can have at least three effects on a Target. Either the probability of the Target decreases (the example already described), increases (an example of an inhibitory connection) or does not change (suggesting no direct connection). Similarly, a Positive Manipulation can also affect the Target positively (in facilitating connections), negatively (in inhibitory connections), or have no effect. Experiments cannot converge on a precise causal hypothesis if they reveal conflicting facilitating and inhibiting relationships. The best they can do is tell us that *A mysteriously* affects *B*. The discernment of different kinds of causal relations is, of course, based on a finer-grained analysis of the outcomes of Single Connection Experiments than simply detecting whether there is an "effect" or "no effect." To sort relationships into inhibitory and facilitating, we must at least distinguish between Connection Experiments that show an increase in the probability of the Target phenomenon (Target-Increase Experiments), those that show a decrease (Target-Decrease Experiments), and those that show no effect in the particular experimental context (Null-Target Experiments). In MCC, experiments that test predictions of enhanced learning, memory, motivation, attention, and so forth (Target-Increase Experiments), are considered to be especially meaningful: it is far easier to break a complex system than to improve it.

As we have cautioned earlier, we must also always keep in mind that the outcomes of experiments may be contingent on their context. Changes in experimental parameters may make the difference between a Null-Target, Target-Increase, or Target-Decrease result. However, with the proper controls and a careful eye for detail, the same manipulations should result in the same effects.

In the absence of temporal information (e.g., Agent *A* changes and *then* we observe a change in Target *B*), it can be difficult to tell from Non-Intervention Experiments alone whether a phenomenon is an Agent or a Target. Without information from manipulation experiments, we may be left to simply note the presence or absence of a correlation. When variables are correlated, they can be either positively correlated (e.g., more *A* leads to more *B*) or negatively correlated (e.g., less *A* leads to more *B*). Otherwise, variables are uncorrelated. We call these different kinds of experiments, by outcome, Positive Correlations, Negative Correlations, and Null-Correlations.

7. A USEFUL TOOL

The scheme just introduced for classifying outcomes across the three kinds of Single Connection Experiment suggests an important heuristic for assessing the reliability of a proposed causal connection. Importantly, this scheme reflects current widespread implicit and explicit practices in Molecular and Cellular Neuroscience. It is also our first explicit principle of Integration. We call this the Convergent 3, and it is based on the following prediction: Assuming that all three kinds of Connection Experiments have been used to test a causal hypothesis, $A{\rightarrow}B$, and assuming that all three kinds of experiments consistently show their predicted effect, subsequent experiments are unlikely to overturn the $A{\rightarrow}B$ hypothesis. In a nutshell, we should bet on the reliability of causal hypotheses that have survived a complete Convergent 3 Analysis. They should be more reliable or stable than those that do not pass a complete Convergent 3 Analysis. However, it does not follow that causal hypotheses that do not (yet) meet the Convergent 3 criteria are false. For example, technical problems in performing some experiments may be the reason for an apparent lack of complete Convergent 3 convergence. In general, neuroscientists working in Molecular and Cellular Cognition (and in other fields that use molecular biology tools) judge such incompletely justified hypotheses as less trustworthy than hypotheses supported by a complete Convergent 3 analysis. The history of neuroscience could be used to test this hypothesis, and the outcomes of such studies could have serious consequences for how practicing neuroscientists make future experimental choices. We'll develop this hypothesis in more detail in later chapters.

8. THE MOLECULAR DANCE

Considered together, the 1992 experiments supported the hypotheses that CaMKII activation affects LTP (CaMKII activation→LTP), CaMKII activation affects Spatial Learning and Contextual Learning (CaMKII activation→Learning), and possibly, CaMKII activation→LTP→Learning. The 1992 experiments were a hook that stuck because they turned out to be useful in testing hypotheses onto which later evidence converged. Or so we hypothesize. To attempt to explain this transformation in terms of the Convergent 3, we need a better grasp on the molecular mechanisms of CaMKII activation. We will start with a series of Identity Experiments, which, as we already described, determine the properties that characterize an individual phenomenon and distinguish it from others.

As Lisman speculated years ago, CaMKII is thought to be capable of storing a biochemical "memory" of its activation (Lisman and Goldring, 1988). This kinase has evolved a number of molecular strategies for its activity to persist long after the increases in postsynaptic calcium fade away. For example, CaMKII can trap the very molecules needed for its activation (calmodulin loaded with calcium). Additionally, the kinase can phosphorylate itself (autophosphorylation). During autophosphorylation, a particular segment of the protein's amino acid structure, a threonine residue in position 286 (Thr286), takes on a phosphate group that acts like an on switch, allowing the kinase to be active even after calcium concentrations have returned to basal levels and calmodulin has become detached. The large phosphate group replaces the calmodulin molecule to keep the kinase domain unencumbered by structural interference from its regulatory domain (for a review of CaMKII, *see* Wayman et al., 2008).

In addition to the Thr286 on-switch, CaMKII also has an off switch. Autophosphorylation at two threonine residues in positions 305 and 306 prevents further interactions with calmodulin, so that kinase molecules phosphorylated at either of these two amino acids can no longer be activated by calmodulin. It is possible that this autophosphorylation event prevents recently activated kinase molecules from repeatedly being turned on by continued synaptic stimulation. (*See* Fig. 4.3).

Recall that according to Lisman's model, CaMKII's capacity to serve as a memory molecule would depend on its sustained activation following synaptic activity. Autophosphorylation at Thr[286] and the resulting persistent kinase activity provides a mechanism for how the initial activation of the kinase, by way of a brief increase in postsynaptic calcium through activated NMDA receptors, could

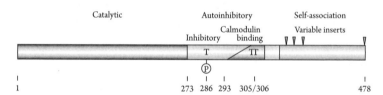

Figure 4.3 The primary structure of the CaMKII protein reveals three functional domains: catalytic, autoinhibitory, and self-association. The catalytic domain makes it possible for CaMKII to phosphorylate other molecules. The self-association domain makes it possible for multiple CaMKII subunits to link together to form a holoenzyme. The variable inserts are sites where different CaMKII isoforms (e.g., α-CaMKII vs. β-CaMKII) differ in amino acid sequences from each other. By phosphorylating itself at 305/306, CaMKII is autoinhibited. Phosphorylation at 286 prevents autoinhibition of CaMKII and puts CaMKII in a persistently active state (Lisman Schulman, and Cline 2002).

result in longer-lasting biochemical changes with a potential impact on synaptic function.

Combining this minimal understanding of CaMKII's structure and function with our analysis of causal effects enables us to articulate the limitations and insights of the evidence from the 1992 experiments. The key insight was that some α-CaMKII event is required for normal synaptic plasticity, providing evidence that α-CaMKII is at least part of a background condition for LTP and learning. However, because these experiments disrupted any activity mediated by α-CaMKII in the knockout mutant mice, they could not reveal the specific CaMKII activity that causally affects learning and LTP. Perhaps, rather than a specific cause, α-CaMKII is like oxygen to learning—necessary for memory in the way that life depends on oxygen, but contributing nothing in terms of specific mnemonic processes. This interpretation can get some traction from the fact that α-CaMKII composes 20% of all synaptic protein! Why have such high levels of a regulatory protein? Could this kinase simply provide part of the structural integrity of the synapse and have no other, more specific causal role in learning and memory? Evidence for the α-CaMKII activation→LTP→learning hypothesis would become stronger if a Non-Intervention Experiment showed that its functional states (e.g., autophosphorylation) change with LTP and learning, and if a Positive Manipulation that increases the levels of the kinase also resulted in enhanced LTP and learning.

9. OBSERVING WITHOUT TOUCHING

The Lisman model offered a hypothesis of features of a memory molecule. CaMKII's action at the synapse had some of these features, and the 1992 experiments showed that CaMKII does *something* to affect learning and LTP. Yet one might still wonder whether CaMKII does what Lisman's model proposed. The 1992 experiments alone do not speak to this. At a minimum, Non-Intervention Experiments would have to be performed to at least confirm that CaMKII autophosphorylation takes place during LTP and learning,

Non-Intervention Experiments measure correlations between phenomena without directly manipulating the hypothesized cause or effect. We were all drilled in our early science training with the truism that "correlation does not prove causation," but it is equally important to note that correlation is a necessary component of testing a causal mechanism. So Non-Intervention Experiments, taking place under biologically realistic circumstances, are necessary to make an integrated experimental case for a hypothesized causal connection.

Non-Intervention Experiments are performed within a specific background context, such as during LTP induction or contextual conditioning. They of course involve experimental manipulations— for example, electrodes to measure LTP in hippocampal slices, a conditioning chamber to measure contextual conditioning—but they omit manipulations intended to change the activation state or probability of the hypothesized causal agent. In considering the hypotheses that CaMKII activation→LTP and that CaMKII activation→Spatial Learning and Contextual Learning, the agent in question is CaMKII activation. We need to see an effect on LTP or learning as that effect is caused by CaMKII's functions.

To test the hypotheses that CaMKII→LTP and that CaMKII→Learning, neuroscientists designed experiments to determine whether behavioral training capable of triggering learning activates CaMKII and whether presynaptic activity sufficient to induce LTP also activates CaMKII. Finding that these two events (i.e., behavioral training and LTP induction) are accompanied by

CaMKII activation supported the hypothesis that CaMKII activation is part of the cause for LTP induction and learning.

A number of studies throughout the 1990s investigated correlations between LTP induction and α-CaMKII activation. As part of a broader study in 1997, Andres Barria and colleagues published a paper indicating that α-CaMKII activation increases when the probability of LTP induction increases (Barria et al., 1997). To measure α-CaMKII activation, Barria used an antibody that binds specifically to α-CaMKII activated by phosphorylation at Thr^{286}. The antibody enabled activated α-CaMKII to be quantified from an extract of hippocampus tissue and to then be compared to control extracts in which LTP was not induced. Barria's Non-Intervention results converged with the α-CaMKII 1992 Negative Manipulation results, at least for the CaMKII activation→LTP induction causal hypothesis. Could CaMKII activation also be correlated in Non-Intervention Experiments with various forms of learning?

One year before Barria's findings were published, Soon-Eng Tan and Keng-Chen Liang found changes in calcium calmodulin-dependent CaMKII activation levels as rats were trained on the water maze task over 5 days (Tan and Liang, 1996). Activated CaMKII phosphorylates syntide2, making it possible to measure CaMKII activation as a function of syntide2 phosphorylation. The higher the level of phosphorylated syntide2, the higher the level of CaMKII activity.[3] They trained their rats on the standard Morris water maze task. Once a rat completed the training, its hippocampus was removed, and syntide2 phosphorylation was measured. No significant changes in total CaMKII levels were observed in any of their experiments. However, as escape latencies decreased over the course of daily training trials, indicating learning, levels of *activated* (calcium calmodulin-independent)

CaMKII activity in hippocampus tissue increased. The higher the percentage of CaMKII activity in hippocampus tissue, the lower the animal's escape latency in the hippocampus-dependent Morris task—or, theoretically, the better the animal's spatial learning and memory.

Interestingly, Tan and Liang also showed in the same paper that an inhibitor of CaMKII, KN-62, impaired spatial learning. Thus, their complete study combined a Negative Manipulation Experiment with the Non-Intervention Experiment described above. They concluded that "the activation of CaM-kinase II [*sic*] in the hippocampus is not only correlated to the degree of spatial training on the Morris water maze, but may also underlie the neural mechanism subserving spatial memory." It is important to note, however, that Tan and Liang's experiments could not distinguish between the different types of CaMKII in the hippocampus. These different kinase isoforms are thought to be part of molecular complexes with coordinated activity, and α-CaMKII is by far the most abundant CaMKII isoform in the hippocampus. Nevertheless, the changes measured in these experiments conceivably could have come from other CaMKIIs (e.g., β-CaMKII).

Without ever manipulating CaMKII levels experimentally, Barria's and Tan's Non-Intervention Experiments provided evidence for the model that activation of CaMKII is a cause for LTP and learning. Activation of the kinase was predicted by the Lisman model and was prevented in the knockout mice and by the drug that Tan and Liang used. It now remained to be shown whether a Positive Manipulation of CaMKII could be used to affect learning and LTP—the third form of convergent experimental evidence needed to satisfy the Convergent 3 hypothesis.

10. POSITIVELY COMPLEX

Molecular biologists can take advantage of the regulatory properties of promoters (sequences of DNA that determine where and
when genes are expressed) to control the expression of genes of
interest. To increase α-CaMKII levels in neurons, in 1995 Mark
Mayford in Eric Kandel's laboratory isolated the α-CaMKII promoter and used it to express an extra copy of a mutant α-CaMKII
gene (Bach et al., 1995; Mayford et al., 1995). At first glance, this
manipulation may be considered a Positive Manipulation (i.e., it
resulted in more CaMKII). However, the kinase overexpressed
was incapable of normal regulation; it could not be turned off.
This "run-away" transgenic kinase was capable of phosphorylating and therefore disrupting the normal regulation of the endogenous CaMKII function. Thus, by introducing a constitutively
active kinase, Mayford and colleagues carried out a Negative
Manipulation of kinase regulation. Their transgenic mice had hippocampal LTP and hippocampal-dependent learning deficits, a
result consistent with the idea that CaMKII regulation is critical for
these two phenomena. Interestingly, long-term depression (LTD)
seemed to be favored over LTP in these transgenic mice (Mayford
et al., 1995), another possible reason for the learning deficits of
these transgenic mice.

In experiments published just a year later (1996), Mayford and
colleagues introduced inducible transgenic methods to neuroscience research. They used a novel transgenic approach to control
when their runaway kinase was expressed. Mayford and colleagues
found that they could reverse the LTP and learning deficits caused
by their runaway α-CaMKII simply by turning off its expression
in adult mice (Mayford et al., 1996). Thus, disrupting kinase function during development could not have caused LTP and learning

deficits in α-CaMKII mutants, as it had been reasonably suspected. Had this been the case, Mayford would not have been able to reverse these learning deficits simply by turning off the mutant kinase in adult mice prior to training. The mutant kinase was under the regulation of a promoter system (tet-off system) that could be turned off by the addition of a tetracycline analog (doxycycline). (*See* Fig. 4.4.) The Mayford experiments added to the growing evidence that disruption of α-CaMKII function affected LTP and learning, but they did not speak to the effects of increased levels of the *normal* kinase.

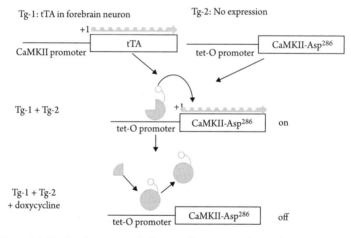

Figure 4.4 To develop mice with the tet-off system, two lines of transgenic mice are made: Tg-1 and Tg-2. Tg-1 receives the gene for the tetracycline transactivator (tTA), placed under the control of the CaMKII promoter so that it will only be expressed in the forebrain, where CaMKII is abundant. Tg-2 receives the modified CaMKII gene linked to the tet-O promoter. Tg-1 and Tg-2 mice are then mated to produce Tg-1 + Tg-2 mice. In these mice, tTa will be produced when wildtype CaMKII is produced, and tTa will induce transcription of the mutant CaMKII by binding to the tet-O promoter. Introducing doxycycline (a tetracycline analog) will prevent tTa from binding to the tet-O promoter, turning off expression of the runaway form of CaMKII.

In 2003, Huimin Wang and colleagues in Joe Tsien's lab overexpressed the mutated gene for a α-CaMKII protein that appeared to function normally (Wang et al., 2003). Nevertheless, they reported abnormal CA1 plasticity and deficits in learning in these mutants. Although LTP seemed generally enhanced in their mutant mice, long-term depression (LTD) was either impaired or enhanced depending on the frequency used to trigger plasticity in the mutant slices. Although high-frequency stimulation usually induces LTP, low-frequency stimulation triggers LTD. In these mutants, the relation between the frequency of stimulation and synaptic change was profoundly altered. The whole S-like curve characterizing this relation was shifted to the right in the mutants, revealing severely abnormal synaptic plasticity.

To control when their overexpressed kinase was activated, they used a powerful technique developed by Kevan Shokat to re-engineer the ATP-binding site of kinases (Bishop et al., 2000). As mentioned above, kinases need ATP to phosphorylate substrates. Shokat's re-engineered ATP-binding site could also bind a specially designed chemical inhibitor. This inhibitor was constructed to be exquisitely specific to the mutant kinase.

When given to the transgenic mice expressing the engineered kinase, the inhibitor turns off the transgenic kinase without disrupting normal kinases or supposedly having any other effects. To drive the expression of their engineered kinase in transgenic mice, Wang used Mayford's α-CaMKII promoter. They showed that their transgenic kinase was expressed in many of the same brain regions and cell types as wildtype or endogenous α-CaMKII. They also showed unequivocally that their mutant mice had higher levels of α-CaMKII than normal.

These were very carefully executed experiments using novel and ground- breaking techniques, but their results were complex and unexpected: The mutation resulted in abnormal plasticity across a wide range of stimulations, and not surprisingly learning was also impaired. Nevertheless, at certain frequencies of stimulation, LTP was enhanced in the mutants. Were the authors not so careful and thorough, the findings could have been very misleading. Without information about a broad range of stimulation frequencies, the findings would have suggested that increases in αCaMKII enhance LTP but cause deficits in learning.

What was causing the learning *deficits* in these transgenic mice? Could this have been caused by the abnormal synaptic plasticity (e.g., deficits in LTD) that these authors identified? Alternatively, were Wang and colleagues' behavioral results an artifact of the overexpression of α-CaMKII, which may drive this kinase to phosphorylate and affect the function of proteins that it never normally contacts? Beyond any potential abnormal functions of the overexpressed kinase, it is also possible that because the manipulations described were not specific to the hippocampus, they affected many other brain regions. Could changes in these other regions account for the learning deficits?

Interestingly, Dave Poulsen, Michael Babcock and colleagues in 2007 showed that a subtler and more specific Positive Manipulation of α-CaMKII results in learning enhancements in rats (Poulsen et al., 2007). Poulsen and colleagues used a virus to overexpress the α-CaMKII gene specifically in the hippocampus of adult rats. They showed that this manipulation improved performance in the water maze. In other experiments, Pierre-Marie Lledo in Roger Nicoll's laboratory in 1995 had shown that delivering CaMKII to the postsynaptic cell with a recording pipette was sufficient to induce a potentiation in CA1 hippocampal slices that looked at lot like LTP (Lledo et al., 1995). Together these last two sets of experiments showed that increases in the levels of CaMKII are sufficient to trigger the potentiation of CA1 synapses and that small, directed increases can (under certain circumstances) enhance learning. But, which experimental results should we trust? The results from the Tsien laboratory suggesting that increases in CaMKII lead to abnormal synaptic plasticity and learning or those just cited seemingly demonstrating the opposite result? Could the differences result from the very different conditions used, from the deficits in LTD in Wang's mutant mice, or from some other variable? The uncertainty in interpreterting the results of individual experiments is the key reason why convergence among a large number of *different* experiments is important.

11. CONFLUENCE AMONG EXPERIMENTS

Rationally planning future research requires that we bet on the reliability of prior results. Convergent evidence justifies those bets. Taking an overview of the experiments we have described in this chapter helps us to see the pattern of convergence.

The evidence that we have described (Table 4.1) supports the general idea that normal α-CaMKII function is needed for hippocampal-dependent learning and CA1 synaptic plasticity, including LTP. Those experiments showed that deleting α-CaMKII, disrupting its regulation, and overexpressing it (perhaps abnormally) leads to deficits in LTP and learning, whereas subtle and more specific increases in its levels can enhance the probability of LTP and learning. The Negative Manipulations yielded Negative Target results, whereas some of the Positive Manipulations yielded Positive Target results. Importantly, Non-Intervention Experiments suggested that increases in

Table 4.1 A Collection of Experiments that Together Satisfy the Convergent 3 Heuristic

Hypothesis	Positive Manipulation	Negative Manipulation	Non-Intervention
CaMKII→LTP	+Target (Lledo et al., 1995)	–Target (Silva et al., 1992a)	+ Correlation (Barria et al., 1997)
CaMKII→L&M	+Target (Poulsen et al., 2007)	–Target (Silva et al., 1992b)	+ Correlation (Tan and Liang, 1996)

+Target = The outcome of the experiment was an increase in the probability of LTP or Learning & Memory.

–Target = There was decrease in the probability of these target outcomes.

+Correlation = Non-Intervention Experiments showed that probability of LTP and Learning & Memory goes up and down as the probability of CaMKII activation goes up and down.

CaMKII activity are correlated with increases in synaptic potentiation and with learning. Importantly, the inducible transgenic experiments from the Kandel and Tsien laboratories did show that manipulations of CaMKII affect LTP and learning. Although we are left with many unanswered questions, a Convergent 3 analysis of all of the evidence tells us that LTP and learning likely depend causally on CaMKII activation.

And yet, the evidence we've discussed has clear limitations. It tells us little about *how* α-CaMKII does what it does, which will of course be relevant for driving further explorations of its role in synaptic plasticity and learning. Is there a triggering causal relation between α-CaMKII and LTP and between α-CaMKII and learning, or is this kinase simply a background condition for these two phenomena? The totality of convergent evidence seems to suggest that this kinase is part of a trigger for LTP and learning. But most neuroscientists would agree that definitive evidence for these hypotheses would depend on additional experiments, which we have not discussed yet. These other experiments provide mechanistic details for the mediating steps between CaMKII activation and LTP and between CaMKII activation and learning. In other words, the strength of the evidence for these other causal connections contributes to the strength of evidence for the causal connections among CaMKII, LTP, and LEARNING. Knowing how CaMKII modulates LTP causally helps to decide whether CaMKII definitely modulates LTP causally.

12. THE EVER-PRESENT COMPLEXITY OF NATURE

The 1992 α-CaMKII transgenic experiments provided evidence for the hypothesis that synaptic molecules with a role in LTP may also be critical for learning and memory. The interdisciplinary strategy introduced in those experiments had considerable potential and scientific appeal because it provided a way to study molecular and cellular mechanisms of behavior with a plethora of Positive and Negative Manipulations of any one of the thousands of genes expressed in the brain. And yet we must be cautious. Changes in one gene affect the expression of many others, the proteins encoded by these genes have complex interactions with many others, and the cells that express the mutant genes are themselves connected with many others in multiple brains regions. Could this mind-bending complexity muddy attempts to connect the function of single genes with the properties of brain regions, much less with the behavior of mutant mice? It is easy to be seduced by the latest shiny tool, by a flashy finding hot off the press, but we must remember that even the simplest of experiments confronts the ever-present complexity of nature. In the next chapter, we will explore the provocative idea that the only perfect experiments are those that we do not understand. We will also argue that the complexity and uncertainty of individual experiments, and the sheer magnitude of the experimental record, demands that we develop novel strategies to determine what is known, what is uncertain, and what may be worth knowing.

[5]

RULING OUT THE
PROBABLE TO ARGUE
FOR THE POSSIBLE

1. HEDGING THE CONVERGENT 3

In the previous chapter, we introduced the first of our Integration principles: the Convergent 3 Analysis. Among molecular and cellular neuroscientists, and perhaps other molecular and cellular biologists, there seems to be a general, implicit consensus that causal hypotheses supported by all three types of evidence represented in the Convergent 3 are more trustworthy than those supported by fewer types of convergent evidence. Convergent 3 analyses simply try to make these implicit commitments explicit. Reasons for this consensus are not difficult to grasp. Each kind of Connection Experiment has the potential to provide unique information about a causal system, and each has the potential to accommodate the others' weaknesses. However, it has not yet been formally demonstrated that findings that satisfy the Convergent 3 are more reliable than findings with only partial support. So, at present we offer only the hypothesis that it does and some considerations of why that hypothesis is reasonable.

Although important, the Convergent 3 is only one of several Integration principles used in molecular and cellular cognition (*see* Fig. 5.1). Consistency in results is also critical. A neuroscience hypothesis supported by evidence from each type of experiment in the Convergent 3 is not accepted if there is an abundance of conflicting results in the published record. Fulfilling the requirements of the Convergent 3 by picking and choosing among the data would defeat the purpose of using this heuristic. First and foremost, the Convergent 3 is a tool, and as such, it can be easily misused.

In his influential book "The Double Helix," which describes the discovery of the structure of DNA, Jim Watson acknowledged that large bodies of data always contain inconsistencies and seeming contradictions. Technical problems and unexpected complexities can lead to results that at least on the surface contradict large amounts of data. But, how much contradiction is too much? Do we resolve these contradictions by weighing evidence for or against a given hypothesis and then choosing a winning side? What are the criteria for deciding whether a body of data supports or refutes a given hypothesis? These are all interesting and important questions that systematic studies of science could help to resolve and that may affect how we judge the usefulness of the Convergent 3 and other rules of Integration that we will introduce later in the book. Misinterpretation of results is another problem that could lead to problems with using the Convergent 3. Misinterpreted experiments can create erroneous contradictions in a data set and consequently give the appearance that the Convergent 3 hypothesis failed. Misinterpreted experiments can also provide an illusion of convergence.

The process of determining whether the requirements of the Convergent 3 hypothesis have been met (i.e., the use of Convergent 3 analysis) is complex and it depends considerably on an understanding of the system being tested. For example, at first glance

Mayford's influential 1995 and 1996 α-CaMKII experiments may seem like examples of Positive Manipulations of α-CaMKII activation, as his experimental manipulations increased the levels of active α-CaMKII in the brain. However, his transgenic manipulations increased the levels of a kinase that lacked the domains critical for α-CaMKII regulation. More importantly, because the multiple stages of α-CaMKII regulation are controlled by phosphorylation, the lack of regulation of the constitutively active transgenic kinase also disrupted the regulation of the endogenous kinase. A superficial reading of this work, however, may have ignored the lack of regulation of the transgenic kinase. Consequently, it would have concluded that because overexpression of αCaMKII leads to deficits in LTP and learning, this kinase has an inhibitory relation to these two phenomena (i.e., more CaMKII → less LTP and less Learning). This misinterpretation of Mayford's experiments would predict that deleting the kinase (Negative Manipulation) would result in enhancements in both LTP and learning and that during LTP or learning, one should see decreases in the activity of this enzyme (Non-Intervention Experiments). As we saw in the previous chapter, these predictions would be in conflict with a considerable number of published Negative Manipulation and Non-Intervention Experiments. Further, as we saw in the previous chapter, mild increases in normal α−CaMKII (Positive Manipulations) did result in LTP and learning enhancements. Mayford's α-CaMKII experiments are more appropriately classified as Negative Manipulation experiments, within a Convergent 3 Analysis of the CaMKII activation → LTP and CaMKII activation → Learning causal hypotheses.

Troubles with the interpretation of results and troubles with contradictions are related matters. Sometimes the appearance of a contradiction is actually the result of misinterpretation. Other times, the consistency of support on offer for a hypothesis is only

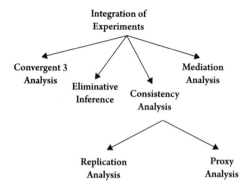

Figure 5.1 A schematic overview of Integration. This chapter will include discussions of the Convergent 3 Analysis and Eliminative Inference. Future chapters will include discussions of Consistency Analysis and Mediation Analysis.

evident when a misinterpretation of data is corrected. In this chapter, we will focus on experimental interpretation itself and we will expand our framework to include other forms of Integration.

Integration Analyses are the routines used implicitly or explicitly by neuroscientists in the evaluation of groups (large or small) of experiments. Integration efforts are most visible in the introductions and conclusions of every research paper. They are at the basis of every published review and play a central role in framing and organizing research proposals. In the previous chapter, we focused on application of the Convergent 3 analysis as a form of Integration. In this chapter, we will focus on Eliminative Inference Analysis. We will leave Consistency Analysis and Mediation Analysis for later chapters.

2. THE DANGER OF A LITTLE LEARNING

In the early days of molecular and cellular cognition research, Richard Morris and Mary Kennedy published a commentary on the 1992 αCaMKII results (Morris and Kennedy, 1992). They expressed both admiration and skepticism. They titled their article, "The Pierian Spring" and opened it with a famous quote from Alexander Pope's *An Essay on Criticism*: "A little learning is a dangerous thing."

The proverbial danger Morris and Kennedy were warning about was the conclusion that the 1992 CaMKII studies had uncovered a component of the mechanism of learning and memory. Morris and Kennedy argued that many potential confounding factors made such a conclusion premature. Side effects of the genetic manipulations or subtleties of the psychological tests used might explain the α-CaMKII results just as well as the hypothesis that the learning deficits of the mutant mice were the result of diminished α-CaMKII function in hippocampal neurons. Morris and Kennedy made a good case for caution while encouraging a sense of urgency in those interested to learn not just whether α-CaMKII affects LTP and learning, but *how* it does this. As a seasoned behavioral neuroscientist, Morris knew of the need to moderate enthusiasm for the results of experiments of cognitive mechanisms. He had learned first-hand how treacherous the integrated study of physiology and behavior could be.

Implicitly, what Morris and Kennedy were urging was nothing less than commitment to Convergent 3 Analysis. When they wrote "The Pierian Spring" criticism, only the results of one Negative Manipulation experiment supported the link between α-CaMKII and either LTP or learning. Caution was certainly warranted.

The Convergent 3 Analysis provides neuroscientists with a rule of thumb for gaging the robustness of Connection experiment results, and thus the reliability of their causal hypotheses. Ideally, causal hypotheses should be supported by all three types of Connection Experiments. In addition, a systematic and thorough elimination of alternative hypotheses or explanations for the results—an Integration process called Eliminative Inference—is also critical. At any given time, some alternative explanations will be more prominent than others. If we can rule out those prominent alternatives, then we can reduce the chances of erroneous interpretations affecting future experiments. The goal of Eliminative Inference is to nip dead-end research paths in the bud, before considerable time and money are invested on them. As a start, a science of experiment planning would benefit greatly from systematic documentation of likely confounds and the identification of experiments that have ruled out those confounds. The more experiment types (Positive and Negative Manipulations, as well as Non-Interventions) are performed to test a given causal connection, the higher the efficiency of the process of eliminating alternative explanations. Morris and Kennedy's concerns with the initial hype surrounding the 1992 α-CaMKII results were justified. Without the extensive body of experiments that followed those 1992 results, it would be unclear whether α-CaMKII was causally related to either LTP or learning. There were simply too many alternative explanations that the initial findings had not addressed. In 1992 the process of Eliminative Inference concerning the possible connection between α-CaMKII, LTP, and learning had just started. This process was made famous by Sherlock Holmes in the "The Sign of the Four": "When you have eliminated the impossible, whatever remains, *however improbable, must be the truth.*"

3. WHODUNIT?

The convergent evidence supporting α-CaMKII's role in LTP and learning (reviewed in Chapter 4) was unavailable at the time that

Morris and Kennedy's commentary was published. Because the 1992 CaMKII experiments were new, their results were vulnerable. Morris and Kennedy's commentary focused on three shortcomings. The first concern, already mentioned in the previous chapter, was that the α-CaMKII manipulation may have affected post-natal development of the mutant mice, suggesting that developmental changes, and not α-CaMKII function in adult mice, could have been responsible for the impairments in LTP and learning.

The second shortcoming was that the α-CaMKII knockout mice lacked the kinase not only in the hippocampus but also in neocortex, striatum, amygdala, and other structures where neurons normally express this protein. The disruption of kinase function in these other structures complicates the proposed explanation that hippocampal-dependent memory had been affected *per se*. Perhaps, the deficits in spatial learning and contextual conditioning of the mutant mice were the result of deficits in these other structures. The methods used in the 1992 α-CaMKII papers brought unprecedented molecular specificity and experimental flexibility into neuroscience. However, these advances came with a price. The early genetic engineering methods lacked the desired developmental and neuroanatomical specificity. In 1992, one could not yet "turn on" the genetic modification specifically after normal developmental processes had occurred, nor could one target the modification to a specific brain region.

A third shortcoming pointed out by Morris and Kennedy was that the α-CaMKII knockout mice trained on the hidden platform task might have performed poorly not because they had spatial learning deficits but because they were relying on a different search strategy than their non-mutant counterparts. The fact that the α-CaMKII mutation also disrupted another very different hippocampal-dependent task (contextual conditioning) helped

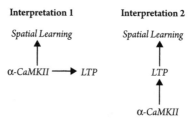

Figure 5.2 Two alternative representations of the 1992 CaMKII experimental results. In Interpretation 1, CaMKII does not affect spatial learning by affecting LTP but through some other mechanism. In Interpretation 2, CaMKII has its impact on spatial learning in the water maze because of its effects on LTP.

to argue that hippocampal learning was disrupted, but it did not completely defray this criticism. It is important to point out that the initial experiments could not have addressed all of these challenges at once. One paper cannot both open and close a case, especially one reporting experiments in a new area of study. Follow-up studies are always required for more supporting evidence (i.e., Convergent 3 Analysis) and to eliminate alternative explanations (i.e., Eliminative Inference). For example, new techniques had to be used to restrict the genetic manipulation to the hippocampus and to address the possibility of hidden developmental abnormalities.

4. ALTERNATE PATHS

Let us pause for a moment and consider the hypotheses that the 1992 α-CaMKII results suggest. In the simplest scenarios, α-CaMKII could affect LTP and, through LTP, affect hippocampal-dependent learning. This was the hypothesis we discussed earlier in this book: CaMKII→LTP→Learning. Alternatively, α-CaMKII could affect LTP and by some other hippocampal physiological mechanism (e.g., inhibition, excitability) affect learning performance. Both of these scenarios are compatible with the evidence included in the 1992 study (Silva et al., 1992a, 1992b; *see* Fig. 5.2). However, they are not the only possibilities.

Morris and Kennedy' Pierian Spring offered additional alternatives for the behavioral learning and memory deficits of the α-CaMKII mutants: (1) developmental changes induced by the α-CaMKII mutation; (2) disruption of kinase function outside of the hippocampus; and (3) alternative search strategies in the water maze (*see* Fig. 5.3). One particularly interesting feature of these alternatives is that they each discount the value of the LTP impairments in deciding the best interpretation of the 1992 α-CaMKII results. More precisely, these interpretations tell us that the LTP impairments, induced by the genetic mutation, *do not necessarily imply* impairments in learning. They counsel that we remain noncommittal on LTP's role in the story.

Given that in any one experiment we cannot typically measure all relevant variables, it is impossible to simultaneously eliminate all possible confounds in one experimental swoop. Often we are even unaware of potential problems until we expose our results to broader scrutiny. Even worse, attempts to rule out confounds with additional experiments typically introduce new confounds. Therefore, it is crucial to obtain multiple lines of convergent evidence for any one causal hypothesis. Yet in the process of building convergent evidence for or against a given hypothesis, there will often be better and worse bets. Time and money are precious, so we want to investigate the best bets first. In the case of the original 1992 α-CaMKII experiments, to determine the best bets among the possible explanations for the original experimental results, we can look to the experiments we discussed in the previous chapter

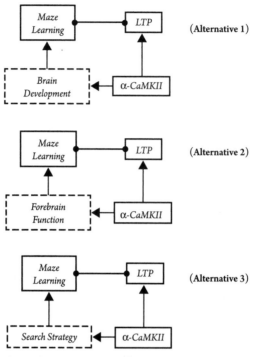

Figure 5.3 Three alternative hypotheses are forwarded in Morris's Pierian Spring. Edges with dots at the ends identify interactions that are suspected—that is, there may be a connection between LTP and task performance.

and consider whether they address the alternative explanations of Morris and Kennedy's Pierian Spring.

Recall that in some of the experiments described in the previous chapter, which followed directly the 1992 studies, mice were engineered with a pharmacologically controllable mutation. Using these inducible transgenic tools, Mayford, Wang, and colleagues were able to show that the effects of their transgenic α-CaMKII manipulations on LTP and learning did not result from developmental changes. Alleviating their adult mutant mice of the overexpressed α-CaMKII returned them to normal learning performance.

Similarly, Liang and Tan's pharmacological disruption of CaMKII function, Poulsen's overexpression of α-CaMKII, and Lledo's electrophysiological experiments showed that this kinase could affect LTP and learning independently of any possible effects on development. These results were described in detail in the previous chapter.

Because in some of Wang's experiments α-CaMKII was only manipulated after training ended, the deficits in the induced mutants also could not be attributed to differences in learning strategies between mutants and controls. The inducible mutants learned with the mutant transgene in the off state and were tested after the mutant transgene had been turned on. Liang and Tan's Non-Intervention Experiments involved no α-CaMKII Manipulations, so neither developmental confounds nor peculiarities of learning strategies induced by α-CaMKII mutations could explain their results. However, Liang and Tan's results did not directly address the possibility that α-CaMKII activation specifically in hippocampal neurons is critical for spatial learning. Before reaching the hippocampus, spatial information is first processed in thalamic and neocortical circuits, and this could contribute to the deficits of the mutant mice. Therefore, it would be preferable if the α-CaMKII mutation were restricted to the hippocampus. This regional specificity would simplify the interpretation of the results. The more specific and well controlled the experiment, the simpler the process of *Eliminative Inference* and, hence, the more reliable the conclusions.

To address the problem of neuroanatomical specificity, Babcock and colleagues used viral vectors to either disrupt or overexpress α-CaMKII specifically in the hippocampus of adult rats. Their experiments (Poulsen et al., 2007) showed that although disruption of α-CaMKII activation specific to the hippocampus led to hippocampal learning deficits, overexpression led to enhancements! It is important to note that their Positive Manipulations used a wild-type kinase and probably resulted in a less robust overexpression of the kinase than Wang's transgenic Positive Manipulation Experiments, where overexpression led to learning deficits. It is likely that the relation between α-CaMKII activity and learning follows the famous, but very common, inverted U-shaped curve: mild increases in kinase activity result in increases in learning, whereas large increases have the opposite effect (*see* Fig. 5.4). Large increases in kinase levels may lead to other effects, such as LTD deficits or ectopic or misplaced phosphorylation events, that interfere with normal learning.

These observations do not speak to all of the alternative explanations for the 1992 findings. Specifically they do not bear on the possibility that CaMKII affects learning by modulating physiological mechanisms other than LTP. Indeed, a number of recent findings have shown that this kinase modulates neuronal excitability

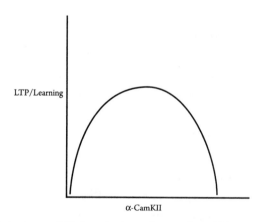

LTP/Learning

α-CamKII

Figure 5.4 An inverted U-shaped relationship might hold between extent of CaMKII activation (x-axis) and LTP and learning (y-axis). To a point, higher levels of CaMKII activation strengthens LTP and learning, but past that threshold higher levels of this kinase will result in progressively weaker LTP and learning.

(Cho et al., 2012)! However, since the publication of the initial α-CaMKII studies, a very large body of data collected with similar genetic, electrophysiological, and behavioral approaches investigated hundreds of genes/proteins in CA1 LTP and showed that this physiological process has a key role in hippocampal-dependent learning. It would be very difficult now to come up with an alternative explanation that could account for all of the data that connects LTP to learning. Similarly, it is highly unlikely that the CaMKII convergent data obtained by several different laboratories, using different pharmacological, transgenic and viral vector approaches, is the result of technical and other artifacts that just happened to be consistent with the LTP/learning hypothesis. Presumably, this kind of coincidence is unlikely. So, although we might still be able to formulate additional alternative explanations for the data, having ruled out the challenges posed by Morris and Kennedy's Pierian Spring, we can more safely conclude that interpretation 2 in Figure 5.2 is a better bet than other interpretations from the full list on offer.

5. TRIPPING ON AP5

After the splash of their 1986 *Nature* paper, where Morris's group first reported that the NMDA antagonist AP5 impairs LTP and spatial learning (discussed in Chapter 3), they carried out rigorous control experiments. In a series of carefully designed dose–response experiments, Morris's lab compared concentrations of AP5 in the hippocampus with the reduction of dentate gyrus LTP (measured in vivo) and the impairment of spatial learning (Davis et al., 1992). As we described before, Morris and colleagues were able to show that animals with the higher hippocampal concentrations of AP5 had larger deficits in both dentate gyrus LTP and spatial learning.

This was an important finding and a valuable follow up to their 1986 results.

Characterizing the dose dependency of a drug's effect is the bread and butter of experimental pharmacology, and on the surface the results of these AP5 experiments seemed to considerably strengthen Morris's 1986 *Nature* findings. However, a careful reading of their now classic 1992 paper in the *Journal of Neuroscience* reveals a puzzling observation. An AP5 dose that seemed to be sufficient to block all LTP, measured in vivo in the dentate gyrus, had only a negligible negative effect on spatial learning! If LTP were essential for spatial learning and memory, as Morris and colleagues claimed, then how could a seemingly complete block of hippocampus LTP leave hippocampal learning largely unaffected? Higher concentrations of the NMDA receptor blocker did result in more severe learning deficits, but this could have resulted from nonspecific (off-target) effects of the drug. Every neuroscientist knows that at higher doses drugs have nonspecific effects. The process of Eliminative Inference had to be called into action. Could AP5 be affecting some other process involved in perception, motivation, and so forth?

Morris's concern with this latter possibility led him to address it with a variety of control experiments. In his 1986 paper, for example, he tested rats treated with AP5 in a visual discrimination task that shared many of the demands of spatial learning but did not require hippocampal function. The fact that the AP5-treated rats were able to master this other task suggested that "the spatial deficit is unlikely to be secondary to a gross disturbance of vision, movement, or motivation" (Davis et al., 1992).

Others were quick to point out that the visual discrimination control task is far less demanding than the spatial learning task, and therefore any impairments related to AP5 in "vision, movement, or motivation" were likely to affect spatial learning far more severely than visual discrimination. To make matters worse, in a single authored paper published in 1989 (Morris, 1989), Morris suggested that AP5 delivery in his experiments was not restricted to the hippocampus but, rather, spread to many other areas of the rats' brains. Because NMDA receptors play a critical role in the neurons subserving sensory processing, and because these receptors are known to have numerous other behavioral functions, there was a real possibility that the spatial learning deficits of the AP5-treated rats were caused by blocking NMDA receptor processes in these other areas (e.g., cortical perceptual processes) and not necessarily NMDA receptor-dependent LTP in hippocampal neurons.

Although certainly deserving of further consideration and study, these concerns might have been forgotten quickly were it not for the careful behavioral experiments that Cain and colleagues carried out with NMDA receptor blockers (Cain et al., 1996). Their work reminded neuroscientists that these drugs were initially developed as anesthetics, but their clinical use had to be discontinued because they triggered disturbing hallucinations. Could the spatial deficits that Morris observed in his AP5-treated rats be the result of abnormal changes in sensory perception (hallucinations)? Cain's data were consistent with the hypothesis that the learning deficits of the AP5-treated rats resulted from impairments other than learning. His experiments, as well as Morris's observations (1989), showed that AP5-treated rats display numerous unusual behaviors (Cain et al., 1996). Many of the drugged rats appeared to be ignoring the escape platform altogether, because during training they climbed on and off of it without stopping. Other rats ignored the escape platform even when they bumped into it during training. How could spatial learning be tested in rats that seemed not to care as much as controls about the very goal of the test—namely, escaping the water by staying on the platform? The uncertainty of whether the behavioral impairments of AP5-treated rats in the standard Morris water maze task resulted from the disruption of hippocampal learning mechanisms came to preoccupy the attention of other behavioral neuroscientists who had been initially enthusiastic about Morris's 1986 findings. In other words, the process of Eliminative Inference identified credible alternative explanations for the original AP5 findings.

Nearly 20 years of experiments, and numerous other published papers describing hundreds of other manipulations of LTP and learning, eventually resolved these troublesome concerns. We now have reason to believe that LTP in the dentate gyrus is only weakly linked to spatial learning tested in the classical version of the Morris water maze (cf. Saucier and Cain, 1995; McHugh et al., 2007). Rather, the version of the task that Morris developed and used is more strongly correlated experimentally with LTP in the hippocampal CA1 region. Therefore, rats with profound LTP deficits measured in the dentate gyrus and nearly normal spatial learning may have had nearly normal CA1 LTP (not enough of the drug may have gotten to the CA1 region to block LTP there). With higher concentrations of the drug, however, enough of it may have made its way into the CA1 region and blocked LTP there. This is a reasonable hypothesis that could be tested with current tools.

Morris's pioneering and influential NMDA receptor experiments illustrate a persistent theme in science. The "honeymoon period" that occasionally accompanies a trend-setting discovery is invariably followed by close and intense scrutiny (much of it involving the process of Eliminative Inference) that often results in alternative, less flattering interpretations of the published data. Eventually the glow of novelty, the enthusiasm and promise of ground-breaking experiments, wanes. We are then faced with the truism that every experiment is imperfect and that only convergence of results gleaned from numerous individually imperfect and very different kinds of experiments brings us closer to scientific truth. That realization is a compelling argument for using Convergent 3 analyses when judging the reliability of a set of findings.

6. ELIMINATION AND INVARIANCE

The original AP5 and α-CaMKII results represent a pioneering phase in the history of learning and memory research. Although we currently have conclusive evidence that NMDA receptors and α-CaMKII activation are important components of CA1 LTP mechanisms, and that these CA1 mechanisms are critical for hippocampal learning and memory, these original experiments are no longer regarded as the only platform for supporting that belief. A lot of new evidence has accumulated since those early experiments.

After the process of Eliminative Inference, aimed at evaluating alternative interpretations, we can take greater assurance for accepting a causal hypothesis from a successful Convergent 3 case. When the proper controls have been performed, reasonable alternative explanations considered and tested, we are less likely to be led astray in asserting a causal connection.

Unfortunately, misinterpretation of results is not the only road to irrelevance for Convergent 3 analyses. Consistency of the results is also critical. We must perform exhaustive searches for contradictions if the results of our analyses are to be deemed dependable, and we must consider the epistemic value of those contradictions when we find them. Today's contradictions can be tomorrow's new research opportunities—a discovered contradiction is a valuable opportunity to expand current knowledge. Typically, dealing with a contradiction discovered across experimental results does not require abandoning a whole body of data nor an accepted explanation of them. A contradiction often can be resolved by realizing that a hidden assumption can no longer be trusted and should instead be tested directly. Morris's pioneering experiments and the careful control experiments that followed suggested that LTP in the dentate gyrus is not critical for learning the version of the water maze used in those studies. Those behavioral results, along with the hundreds of other genetic experiments that followed, pointed instead to LTP in the hippocampal CA1 region as central to spatial learning tested in the classical version of the water maze.

So what, then, is the role of LTP in the dentate gyrus? To answer this question, McHugh and colleagues in Susumu Tonegawa's laboratory used an elegant genetic strategy to delete NMDA receptors specifically in the mouse dentate gyrus (McHugh et al., 2007). Although this Negative Manipulation resulted in a loss of NMDA receptor-dependent LTP in that region, learning in the classical Morris's water maze task was unaffected. Rather, McHugh found that NMDA receptor-dependent LTP in the dentate gyrus is required for the animal's ability to distinguish between similar environments (tested in an altered version of Morris' task). McHugh's mutant mice could learn to recognize and navigate in any one environment, but they were unable to distinguish it from another similar environment. These results are consistent with theoretical ideas proposed by Rolls and colleagues that plasticity in the dentate gyrus is critical for "pattern separation" (Treves and Rolls, 1994).

A brilliant mathematician-turned-theoretical neuroscientist, David Courtnay Marr, published a paper in 1971 that introduced many of the ideas still used today to interpret and plan hippocampal experiments (Marr, 1971). Marr proposed that the highly interconnected CA fields of the hippocampus were used to store patterns processed in the neocortex and that during recall this unusual inter-connectivity could be used for reconstructing stored patterns from incomplete inputs, a process known as pattern completion. The capacity of such a storage system is dramatically increased if the overlap among the to-be-stored patterns is reduced, a process called pattern separation.

Thus, results such as those from McHugh and colleagues have now solved many of the mysteries of Morris's initial results. Morris carried out truly visionary experiments (i.e., integrating LTP and learning studies), only in the wrong place (i.e., dentate gyrus) for the behavioral task he used. He obtained the right results (i.e., dentate gyrus LTP does have a role in learning) but with the wrong experiments (i.e., testing the hypothesis that dentate gyrus LTP is involved in spatial learning in the classic version of the task he developed).

Incidentally, more recent experiments have shown that the very same α-CaMKII manipulations affecting LTP in CA1 hippocampus neurons do not disrupt dentate gyrus LTP (Cooke et al., 2006). This finding supports the idea that deficits in the CA1, and not the dentate gyrus, were responsible for the spatial learning abnormalities of the original α-CaMKII mutants. Subsequent research has been kind to the early NMDA receptor/CaMKII results. But luck had no small role in that.

It is easy to be carried away by the excitement of novel scientific work, and NMDA receptor/CaMKII work was truly eye opening. But the price of novelty is always high, as the exploration of unmapped territory with uncertain tools is fraught with the unexpected, the uncertain, and the misleading. Maps of research findings could bring a much needed objectivity not only to the early days of a field but also to its graying years, where large bodies of data overwhelm and disorient practitioners possibly leading to biased views of what is actually represented in the published record. In the next chapter we will shift our emphasis from Convergent 3 Analysis and Eliminative Inference to other processes of Integration that will be critical for deriving research maps, whether computer routines or simply pen and paper are used to generate them.

[6]

RESONATING EXPERIMENTS

1. OCEANS OF EVIDENCE

Adrift on seas of data, we sometimes find ourselves struggling to grasp the implications of findings in our own subfields. So we scale down the problem. Limiting ourselves to a small handful of experimental reports, the triple-footed support of a Convergent 3 analysis at least provides us with some stability. We can wrap our heads around only a handful of papers at a time. So long as the number of experiments and associated confounds stays relatively small, we can use the Convergent 3 and other Integration methods to systematically work through the evidence and make progress.

If there are inconsistencies, failures of replication in the relevant experimental record, or if one or more legs of a Convergent 3 Analysis are weakened by conflicting reports, then the tripod may wobble. Evidence must converge not only within any one subset of experiments (e.g., a published paper) but across the experimental record. Occasional anomalies, resulting from imperfect experiments and faulty assumptions, are to be expected. But when anomalies abound, when the experimental record becomes burdened by the growing weight of contradictory evidence, partial convergence across any chosen subset of experiments no longer inspires confidence in the causal hypothesis.

Finding that the Convergent 3 has been satisfied for a given hypothesis renders it promising. Surviving the crucible of Eliminative Inference makes it stronger still. In contrast, unresolved inconsistencies in the published record weaken hypotheses. The critical point is that in deciding which hypotheses are reliable and which are no longer useful, neuroscientists look for consistency and convergence (or a lack of it) not only in isolated subsets of data but ideally in the entirety of the relevant published record. The goal of this chapter is to expand our framework of Integration to include efforts to search for consistency across experiments. We already introduced in previous chapters to two important processes of Integration (Convergent 3 Analysis and Eliminative Inference). In this chapter we will focus on another Integration process: Consistency Analysis.

2. CONSISTENCY ANALYSIS

When multiple manipulations are directed on the same phenomenon (e.g., a pharmacological and a genetic manipulation), when the same experiment is replicated in a different laboratory, we hope that the effects measured in the experiments are compatible and consistent. In other words, beyond Convergent 3 Analysis and Eliminative Inference requirements, the supporting evidence for a hypothesis must also pass a Consistency Analysis (*see* Fig. 6.1). In the crudest case, which sometimes is the best that we can do at any given time, we design experiments to test whether the findings obtained with one manipulation are confirmed with similar or even identical manipulations. When similar manipulations yield different results, neuroscientists must consider which experiments to trust, which to discount, what the probability of a false—negative or false—positive result might be, and whether there were crucial differences between the conflicting experiments. When there is sufficient consistency across experiments and when Convergent 3 Analysis and Eliminative Inference requirements are satisfied, investigations can move forward with the assurance that a causal link has been established.

We distinguish two kinds of Consistency Analysis commonly carried out in neuroscience: those directed at looking for consistency among experiments with exactly the same protocols (Replication Analysis) and those directed at experiments that study conceptually similar variables (Proxy Analysis). They are both crucial components of testing a causal hypothesis. Neuroscientists recognize that it is crucial that important findings be repeated in multiple laboratories and with different approaches. It is comforting to know that multiple transgenic manipulations and various pharmacological experiments have all shown that deletions of α-CaMKII disrupt LTP and learning. The variety of tools used and

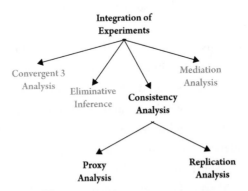

Figure 6.1 Consistency Analysis includes Proxy Analysis and Replication Analysis. In Proxy Analysis, we abstract away from the details of particular experiments and look for consistency. In Replication Analysis, we compare only experiments with the same protocols.

the number of laboratories involved increase our confidence that Negative Manipulations of this kinase actually impair both LTP and learning.

3. THE PROBLEMS WITH MAKING BIG CAUSAL JUMPS

In Chapter 4 we integrated results across three different classes of Connection Experiment, looking at two distinct causal hypotheses: CaMKII activation→LTP and CaMKII activation→Spatial Learning/Contextual Learning. We made the intuitively unlikely look plausible—that knocking out a single gene can meaningfully affect LTP and learning. The challenges of Richard Morris's Pierian Spring, however, forced us to consider alternative hypotheses that also fit the data. Fortunately, we could tap into a large amount of additional data generated after the 1992 CaMKII experiments. The use of Eliminative Inference helped us to reduce the number of plausible interpretations of the results, while our Convergent 3 Analysis provided complementary evidence (Positive Manipulations, Non-Interventions) for those causal connections that went well beyond the Negative Manipulation data in the original 1992 experiments. Based on the experiments we have discussed thus far, it would appear that CaMKII activation is a likely component in the mechanisms of LTP and of learning. However, we did not review all of the evidence that could be considered, nor did we reduce the number of available hypotheses to one.

Two hypotheses that could explain the results of the 1992 CaMKII experiments include Learning←CaMKII→LTP (CaMKII affects LTP and learning separately) and CaMKII→LTP→Learning (CaMKII affects learning by affecting LTP). Suppose that we were interested in evaluating the second hypothesis. What would we have to know to assess its validity?

Does memory depend on LTP? Perhaps surprisingly, neuroscientists do not universally accept the LTP→Learning hypothesis. As of 2013, this hypothesis still evokes considerable skepticism, sometimes accompanied by confused philosophizing about the nature of causation (Lee and Silva, 2009; Neves et al., 2008; Martin and Morris, 2002; Martin et al., 2000). As we first remarked back in Chapter 1, there is much that we do not understand concerning how a cellular phenomenon like LTP could account for the complex behaviors we call "learning and memory." Understandably, neuroscientists are not easily convinced that the evidence available (i.e., the evidence they know about) allows them to confidently make the big jump between LTP and learning. Therefore, resolving the competition between our two CaMKII hypotheses requires clarity about the kind of evidence relevant for assessing the trustworthiness of the hypothesized LTP→Learning link. We propose that the explicit and systematic use of Integration principles may help to resolve this and other similar controversies in neuroscience. It is clear that the implications of the CaMKII activation→LTP causal connection pale in comparison with the LTP→Learning connection. The first concerns one of many biochemical mechanisms that modulate synaptic plasticity, whereas the second is the most studied and most credible mechanism of learning and memory. Therefore, the Integration demands of the LTP→Learning hypothesis certainly exceed those of CaMKII activation→LTP.

We can begin by considering the evidence that we do not need. We do not need a demonstration that LTP is the *only* mechanism linked to memory. We already know that LTP could not alone be responsible for learning. Inhibition and excitability are also very likely to be causally involved in learning and memory. Conceivably, changes in inhibition and excitability could also disrupt or enhance learning, even when those changes do not affect specific measurements of LTP.

Additionally, redundancies are always built into robust complex systems such as the brain. Where such redundancies exist, damage to one component of the system can be compensated for by activities in other components. Thus, to understand the causal structure of neural mechanisms, we should never assume that contributing causes are always *necessary* for their effects, nor do they have to be *sufficient*. Components of complex systems work together with many other components, and in isolation they usually have very little functionality. For example, NMDA receptor activation is a key contributing cause for LTP in hippocampal CA1 pyramidal cells. But NDMA receptors do not do that job alone. They function in concert with AMPA receptors and many other cellular signaling components. Additionally, NMDA receptors are necessary for some forms of LTP, but they are by no means *sufficient* for LTP. Thus, to demonstrate that LTP is causally connected to learning, we do not have to show that this form of synaptic plasticity is *sufficient* for learning. Rather, Convergent 3 Analysis, Eliminative Inference, and Consistency Analyses can be used to evaluate the strength of (or lack of) evidence supporting the hypothesis that LTP is causally connected to learning.

4. SNOWFLAKE EXPERIMENTS

The goal of Consistency Analysis is to determine whether there is coherence among the results of similar Connection Experiments. For example, a Consistency Analysis would determine whether various strategies to carry out a Positive Manipulation of a specific molecule, within the same range of activation, have the same effect on synaptic plasticity. Yet in evaluating the coherence among similar experiments, we must always be cautious not to compare the results of importantly, albeit subtly, different experiments. However subtle, these differences, when properly noted and documented, could be valuable hints that could lead to important insights. As we previously cautioned when describing Convergent 3 Analysis and Eliminative Inference, Consistency Analysis is only a tool, and as such it should be used wisely. A hypothesis with full support from Convergent 3 and Eliminative Inference Analyses should not be lightly discarded because of sporadic anomalies detected during a Consistency Analysis. For example, just because a Negative Manipulation of a given gene in mice affects spatial learning but not contextual conditioning, this does not necessarily mean that the results are contradictory (i.e., the causal link between that gene and learning is unreliable). Although both tasks are hippocampal-dependent, there are differences between them that could help to resolve this apparent contradiction. Of course, a hypothesis is strengthened when a Proxy Analysis detects consistent results across two similar experiments.

Replication Analysis requires exactly the same experimental protocols to be applied to the experiments under consideration. Despite the strictness in the definition of a replication, replications are frequently performed in neuroscience and they are critical for the very fabric of the science. It is important to show that different labs with similar conditions can get similar results. Every time another student learns how to induce LTP in CA1 neurons, he or she is trained using some specific protocol that replicates some prior LTP induction experiment. These training replications are routine but are critical epistemologically. It is impossible to build systematic science on poorly characterized phenomena and undependable techniques.[1] Thus, Replication Analyses are endemic to laboratory science. Replications are critical because their success means that scientists understand the variables critical for a given finding. Without successful replications, it is uncertain whether the declared variables are actually the ones responsible for a given phenomena.

The Negative Manipulation CaMKII experiments we described used two different species, and a variety of molecular manipulations, LTP induction protocols, and learning and memory tasks. By definition, these experiments were not replications, although they shared similar goals and some of the same components. How then can we be certain that these very different experiments carried out in different laboratories were studying the same phenomena (e.g., CA1 LTP, hippocampal learning)? For example, it turns out that there are various forms of CA1 LTP, with different underlying mechanisms. Some forms of CA1 LTP are even NMDA receptor independent. Sometimes what we initially think of as a single phenomenon (e.g., CA1 LTP) is actually several different phenomena (NMDA-receptor dependent LTP, voltage calcium channel-dependent LTP, etc.) with different mechanisms and even different functions. This should always be considered during Integration studies, and it is one of the many reasons why Integration tools, including Consistency Analysis, should never be used blindly and inflexibly.

Neuroscientists often must ignore the fine-grained details of specific experiments, and look for convergence instead among the more rough-grained hypotheses the experiments are designed to investigate. This is the basis of Proxy Analysis. To illustrate this idea, let us consider some Negative Manipulation experiments led by Karl Giese and colleagues in 1998 (Giese et al., 1998). Giese used a point mutation to disrupt α-CaMKII autophosphorylation in neurons and tested the effects on CA1 LTP and water maze learning performance. Recall that the original 1992 Negative

Manipulation experiments used an α-CaMKII knockout mutant (Silva et al., 1992a, 1992b). Despite the fact that both the 1992 and Giese experiments were Negative Manipulations of α-CaMKII function, at a fine-grained level Giese performed very different experiments from the 1992 experiment. But at the level of the general causal hypothesis they were investigating, α-CaMKII$\rightarrow$CA1 LTP$\rightarrow$Spatial Learning, both sets of experiments were Negative Manipulations of α-CaMKII (i.e., they are classified under the same category of a Convergent 3 Analysis). Nevertheless, despite their similarities both sets of experiments were quite different. Giese's experiments, for example, were more selective than the 1992 experiments because they were focused on the function of the domain of α-CaMKII responsible for calcium-calmodulin independent activity. Giese's point mutation deleted a key mechanism in the activation of α-CaMKII, whereas the 1992 knockout experiments eliminated the entire molecule. Despite their drastic differences, the outcomes of both Negative Manipulation experiments confirmed the predictions of the α-CaMKII$\rightarrow$CA1 LTP$\rightarrow$Spatial Learning hypothesis. A Proxy analysis finds that although Giese and colleagues hardly replicated the early work on CaMKII, their results cohered with this earlier work.

Despite the many differences among related experiments, we are capable of identifying relevant similarities. Every experiment is a unique snowflake, but even snowflakes bear important similarities to one another. Sometimes we must use conceptual variables to group experimental variables into comparable—and hopefully cohering—clusters of evidence. When we group differing experiments in this way, and look for consistency among their outcomes, we perform a Proxy Analysis. In evaluating a mechanism's function it is routine—and often experimentally critical—to consider a range of conditions. Robust mechanisms can function under a broad range of input conditions—that's why they're robust. Proxy Analysis is one way neuroscientists determine the robustness of a proposed causal connection. If the connection between LTP and learning is robust, then the connection is likely to manifest itself under a range of different patterns and rates of stimulation. This supposition recommends that we consider a wide range of LTP experiments as a pool of data for assessing the LTP→Learning connection and not confine ourselves to only looking at results from studies that use only one type of LTP manipulation (e.g., a α-CaMKII knockout, pharmacological block of NMDA receptors, etc.) or one kind of LTP induction protocol (100 Hz train; theta-burst pattern, etc.).

5. MIGHT THE HERRING BE RED?

Is LTP part of a mechanism for learning? Or have we been on a wild goose chase for nearly four decades? In 2008 Bliss and colleagues published an opinion piece in a prominent neuroscience journal expressing their tentative views on the evidence, or lack thereof, to support a causal link among LTP, learning, and memory (Neves et al., 2008). Their principal contention was that LTP had yet to be shown *necessary and sufficient* for learning to take place. This claim may well be true. But providing such a demonstration is not the best way to justify causal hypotheses in complex systems like the brain.

To make the case for a genuine causal relationship, Bliss and his collaborators argued that we must be able to implant a false memory by artificially inducing LTP in specific synapses. This demand sets a very high bar for the LTP→Learning hypothesis, far higher than what is typically required for other causal connections in biology. It is instead what one would demand to establish experimentally that learning *just is* LTP: *an identity claim*. Notice that establishing this identity assertion is logically a much stronger demand than demonstrating that LTP is causally central in the network of phenomena responsible for learning. If we wished to justify the identity claim, that LTP *just is* learning, then we would need to show that LTP accounts for all properties of learning. Clearly, this is well beyond our reach, as we do not even know what that would require. Rather, a more realistic (and far more common goal in neuroscience) is to determine whether LTP is *one of the causes* of learning. This is a more modest goal, but for a complex system like the brain, this may be the only reachable goal in the foreseeable future. Additionally, mechanisms other than LTP, including GABA-mediated inhibition (Paulsen and Moser, 1998), have also been implicated in learning and memory, thus ruling out the LTP/ learning identity claim.

How would we determine whether LTP is one of the causes of learning? We propose that we could use the Integration tools we have introduced to sift through the many papers published on the subject and evaluate the weight of evidence for this iconic causal connection. But before we could start on this arduous task, there are a few things that we would need to keep in mind. First, we should focus our analysis on a given class of LTP phenomena (e.g., CA1 LTP) and on a specific type of learning (e.g., hippocampal-dependent learning). Clustering all forms of LTP and all forms of learning would likely muddy up the results. Second, we should not confuse the project of determining whether CA1 LTP, for example, is one of the causes of hippocampal learning with the much bigger project of exactly defining the contribution of CA1 LTP to hippocampal learning. The latter project would require insights into the many causes that mediate between CA1 LTP and hippocampal learning. This is under the auspices of Mediation Analysis, a topic discussed in the next chapter.

Defining how LTP contributes to learning is likely to take decades to complete, whereas we may already have the data required to determine whether CA1 LTP is one of the causes of hippocampal learning. If we distinguish these two—obviously distinct—projects (the *how* and *whether* projects), then we can mount strong arguments for the centrality of LTP in causal mechanisms of some forms of learning and memory without worrying about establishing necessary and sufficient conditions.

6. BURIED TREASURE

The size and complexity of literature focused on iconic causal connections, such as the LTP→Learning link, is a real problem for efforts to extract key conclusions and summary findings. What are we to make of a body of data that seems to include both considerable evidence for and against the LTP→Learning hypothesis? In an attempt to tackle this vexing problem, Lee and Silva (2009) carried out a Consistency Analysis of a specific subset of this vast literature. First, these authors decided to focus on mutant mouse studies that addressed the CA1 LTP→Hippocampal Learning hypothesis, as this area includes most of the data pertaining to the LTP→ Learning hypothesis. Second, they restricted their Consistency Analyses to studies that reported enhancements in hippocampal learning. Most people would agree that although it is easy to break something, it is far harder to make it better. The key question they asked was: Do genetic manipulations that enhance hippocampal learning also enhance CA1 LTP?

Out of the few hundred experimental reports published up until 2008 using mouse hippocampal learning and memory mutants, 33 reported hippocampal learning and memory enhancements. Out of the pool of 33, experimenters had measured LTP in 29 different mutant mice lines. With this list in hand, Lee asked how many of these 29 "smart mice" were also reported to have enhanced LTP in the CA1 region of the hippocampus. There is extensive evidence that this hippocampal region is critical for rodent spatial learning and contextual conditioning, the two most common hippocampal tests used in those 29 reports.

Very few neuroscientists would claim that LTP is the only mechanism of learning and memory. Consequently, one would expect that enhancements induced in other mechanisms could also strengthen learning and memory, without necessarily triggering enhancements in specific measurements of LTP. Indeed, an extensive informal poll taken between 2007 and 2012 of neuroscientists (including the authors) working in this area revealed predictions that 5% to 50% of the "smart mutants" would have enhancements in CA1 LTP (median was approximately 30%). Most of the polled principal investigators working in molecular and cellular mechanisms of learning and memory thought that although a significant fraction of the smart mutants would show enhancements in LTP, the majority would reveal a slew of other physiological phenotypes including changes in inhibition, excitability, and so forth, that would account for the memory enhancements of these mice. Some of our most cynical colleagues (principal investigators of leading learning and memory labs) even predicted that one would find just as many enhancements as deficits in LTP in these "smart" mice! There may be interesting explanations for these varying predictions, and we will discuss them in detail later in this chapter.

The outcome of Lee's Consistency Analysis was utterly unexpected: 27 of the 29 "smart" mouse lines showed enhancements in CA1 LTP! In the two "anomalous" lines, LTP was apparently normal. In one of these two cases, the memory enhancement was observed specifically during "remote" memory tests—that is, tests conducted many days after training. Previous studies had shown that remote spatial and contextual memories depend on neocortical processes (cf. Frankland and Bontempi, 2005). Perhaps future studies in the neocortex will reveal enhanced neocortical LTP in this mutant? In the remaining single "inconsistent" case, the mutation disrupted the alpha 5 GABAA receptor. Blockers of that receptor are known to enhance LTP and learning in rats. Unfortunately, the studies of alpha 5 mutant mice used very strong LTP induction parameters, which may have masked possible enhancements. Nevertheless, the authors of the mouse study reported a small LTP enhancement that did not reach statistical significance. Future studies with milder LTP induction parameters might very well reveal CA1 LTP enhancements even in alpha 5 mutant mice.

It is important to note that the 29 studies reviewed by Lee's Consistency Analysis were carried out by 29 different laboratories, and they used a wide variety of physiological and behavioral conditions. This means that the connection between LTP and learning is very robust and it could not be explained away by the systematic bias of a small group of scientists working with a limited set of misleading electrophysiological and behavioral conditions.

Finally, Lee asked whether the molecular genetic manipulations that resulted in both enhancements in hippocampal learning and CA1 LTP could be organized into coherent signaling pathways. Eleven Positive genetic Manipulations and sixteen Negative genetic Manipulations were responsible for the enhancements in learning and in LTP. Not surprisingly, many of the targeted molecular components were found to be part of the NMDA receptor/CaMKII pathway that we have been discussing. This finding rendered the different molecular enhancements intelligible, in light of the

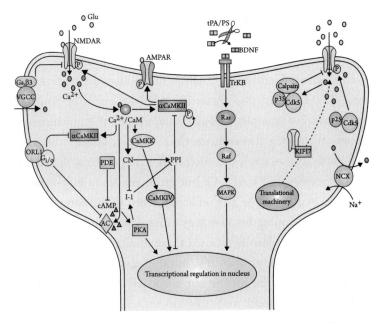

Nature Reviews | Neuroscience

Figure 6.2 Diagram of a dendritic spine. Many of the genetic manipulations of the components shown affect pathways that trace back to the NMDA receptor (NMDAR; upper left corner). Flat-headed arrows represent proposed inhibitory connections. Pointed arrowheads indicate proposed facilitating causal connections. Reprinted with permission from Lee and Silva (2009).

well-supported dependency among NMDA receptors, CaMKII, LTP, and learning. (*See* Fig. 6.2.)

Beyond the implications for LTP and learning of Lee's Consistency Analysis, there is a larger question concerning the considerable discrepancy between the results of the analysis and prevalent views and expectations in the field. Why is it that leading researchers in the field (and the authors were no exception!) thought that only 5% to 50% of the smart mice would also show enhancements in LTP versus the more than 90% result reported in the study?

7. CAUSES AND THEIR MANY CONSEQUENCES

Even a cursory Consistency Analysis of the literature pertinent to the LTP→Learning hypothesis identifies a number of potential confounds. For example, although manipulations that enhance hippocampal learning also enhance CA1 LTP (*see* above), there are well-publicized examples of molecular manipulations that result in enhancements in CA1 LTP but cause deficits in hippocampal learning. In addition to LTP enhancements, these manipulations may disrupt learning because they cause deficits in other mechanisms needed for learning. Could these results be responsible for the misperception of the LTP/learning data discussed above? Could these cases be biasing our collective intuition against the LTP→Learning hypothesis?

Although our discussions have focused so far on single connections between pairs of phenomena (an agent and a target), in reality any one causal connection in neuroscience is nested in a large network of other interacting connections. For example, Grant, O'Dell, and colleagues studied mutant mice lacking PSD95, a synaptic protein. They showed that this mutation enhanced CA1 LTP but caused deficits in hippocampal learning (Migaud et al., 1998). However, the authors noted that the PSD-95 mutation they studied also disrupted LTD and dramatically shifted the balance between these two forms of synaptic plasticity. Because PSD-95 is a structural protein that interacts with many key synaptic components, it is not surprising that the deletion of this protein altered synaptic processes, including LTD, that could be required for learning and memory. In summary, although the mutation of PSD-95 resulted in enhancements in LTP, which by itself would have been expected to enhance learning, it also caused synaptic deficits that could account for the learning deficits of the PSD-95 mutant mice.

Similarly, Fanselow, O'Dell, and colleagues showed that the mutation of the glutamate receptor 2 subunit (GluR2), specifically in the CA1 region, leads to a dramatic enhancement in CA1 LTP but deficits in hippocampal learning (Wiltgen et al., 2010). It turns out that in the absence of GluR2, calcium can enter the cell through glutamate receptors, thus explaining the large potentiation observed in the GluR2 mutant mice. Calcium is an important signaling molecule in synaptic function, and therefore gross deregulation of synaptic calcium signaling would be expected to disrupt learning and memory.

The two examples just described illustrate how manipulations of a single phenomenon (e.g., PSD-95, GluR2) can have multiple effects (e.g., enhancements in LTP, deficits in LTD, disruptions of synaptic calcium, signaling changes, etc.) and that these effects may have opposing consequences in any one given phenomenon of interest (e.g., learning). Consequently, when carrying out a Consistency Analysis, it is important to recognize that a single manipulation may have multiple unintended effects that could impact the interpretation of the results.

A word of caution: Although inconsistencies can be expected to have explanations, they cannot be cursorily brushed aside or ignored. Rather, the evaluation of a hypothesis depends on the painstaking process of systematically weighing each strand of evidence for or against the hypothesis. As this process evolves, and neuroscientists explore the convergences and contradictions in a body of data, hypotheses are discarded or confirmed, and more importantly, if the process is generative, new questions and new insights emerge. In this book, our goal is to articulate a framework and key principles that can be used in this process of carefully evaluating results and deciding where to go next.

8. INTUITION BUGS AND CONSISTENCY ANALYSES

When navigating a large body of data, scientists believe that their intuitions can serve as an internal compass, discarding the trivial, guiding them to important findings, determining what hypotheses the data support and what hypotheses should be discarded. Scientists learn to trust their intuitions. But, is this trust always justified? Considering what is at stake (hundreds of billions of dollars of planned experiments every year), is there a need to objectively test the reliability and efficacy of different aspects of scientific intuition? Although few people would deny the power and usefulness of scientific intuition, might the cognitive processes behind intuition be responsible in certain cases for blatant errors and biases? In other words, without maps, how good are we at navigating large bodies of data?

In a recent book, *Brain Bugs*, Dean Buonomano (2011) explored the extensive body of evidence demonstrating that despite our brains' capacity to solve amazing computational problems, we have appalling weaknesses and shortcomings. Although we can master the obscure and perplexing complex symbology and grammar of a foreign language in months, even elementary algebra baffles us, and we are easy prey to deceptive marketing practices that take advantage of our limited logical skills and distorted motivational systems. Could our limitations, our built-in evolutionary "brain bugs," lead us to systematically commit certain errors when interpreting large bodies of data? Is the current uncertainty concerning whether CA1

LTP is one of the causes of hippocampal learning the result of inconsistent or incomplete data or a consequence of our brain's limitations as an intuitive Integration device? Are logical glitches/fallacies interfering with our ability to discern overall patterns in large and very complex bodies of data? Can we truly navigate the immensity of the published record without the aid of abstract simplifications of the data (i.e., maps)?

9. INTERLUDE ON PHANTOM NEGATIVITY

The results of Lee's 2009 study were both surprising and encouraging. They demonstrated that experimental work on CA1 LTP has not been a diversion in the quest to discover mechanisms of learning and memory. But the lost souls of unpublished results haunt any such analysis. Perhaps, we see consistency only because others have not published—or have not been able to publish—results dissociating LTP from learning. Is there any way to account for, or at the very least investigate, this possibility in a Consistency Analysis?

One might expect, with a hypothesis as seminal as LTP→Learning, that any studies apparently refuting it would attract quite a bit of interest. And indeed, in 1999, a handful of scientists who ran very prominent laboratories, including Per Andersen, Peter H. Seeburg, and Bert Sakmann, published a high-profile study in the journal *Science*, where they reported that an AMPA receptor mutation affecting primarily glutamatergic receptors outside of synapses (GluR A) resulted in deficits in CA1 LTP (Zamanillo et al., 1999). However, the same mutation did not seem to affect spatial learning in the water maze. These results attracted a great deal of attention because they seemed to provide direct evidence that CA1 LTP was not needed for spatial learning. Three years later, however, some of those same authors published another, less well-known paper, where they reported that the deficit in LTP reported was very sensitive to the induction protocol used (Hoffman et al., 2002). The paper showed that some forms of CA1 LTP were actually preserved in the GluR A mutants. Importantly, these studies used stimulation patterns for inducing LTP (theta bursts) that mimic activation patterns seen in vivo during learning. These results of LTP in the GluR A mutants were hardly surprising, as this mutation did not seem to result in a substantial change in glutamatergic synaptic currents.

Setting aside noteworthy exceptions, there may be disincentives for publishing results that go against prevailing dominant hypotheses. There is an understandable bias toward positive results in the study of a novel phenomenon. However, we must not lose sight of the fact that the rewards can be quite high for results that defy prevailing dogma. There are many examples of the importance of paying attention and following up anomalous findings. The barrage of epigenetic findings in every field of biology, including neuroscience, is a good example of this (Levenson and Sweatt, 2005; Egger et al., 2004). In contemporary discussions, "epigenetics" refers to patterns of trait expression that do not result from Mendelian genetic processes per se, but rather are the work of non-genetic (not in the DNA code) mechanisms that control when and where specific genes are expressed. The prevailing dogma was that heritable differences in traits were entirely the result of differences in the genetic code. There would be no field of epigenetics research if the anomalous results of genetic experiments had been ignored and related phenomena (e.g., DNA methylation and histone modification) overlooked.

Although the potential significance of anomalous findings is widely recognized, the risks of studying and publishing anomalous findings, especially when defying convention, should not be underestimated. There are good reasons for this resistance—anomalies in science can be caused by overlooked phenomena or by careless experiments. The stronger the evidence supporting a given hypothesis, the harder it is to convince the scientific community that an important aspect of a strong hypothesis may be wrong. Therefore, researchers pursuing these results can expect their experimental and technical competence to be called into question, their submitted papers rejected, and their grant proposals denied. But in the end, the payoffs can be just as large.

If we wish to increase publication of anomalous results, for the sake of learning the truth about hypothesized neural mechanisms, then we will need to create an infrastructure that reduces these costs to investigators and provides positive career incentives to motivate them to make public their less glamorous data. With the recent arrival of journals like the All Results Journals, devoted to publishing even negative results, we are optimistic that these obstacles can be overcome. In running Consistency Analysis on the results of experiments probing complex systems, anomalous and even negative results can be precious. We must treat them as such.

10. TYING TOGETHER THE CAUSAL NETWORK

It is tempting to conclude that there is an established causal relation between CA1 LTP and hippocampal-dependent learning. But, when the evidential standards used to judge a hypothesis are confused or disproportionate to the task—as are the requirements of necessary and sufficient conditions to establish causal relevance, for example—we will suspend belief indefinitely or possibly buy into a misleading hypothesis. We must be rigorous and firm, yet we must also be reasonable and consistent about the proper demands of causality.

Each of the articles cited in Lee's 2009 study are understandably limited in scope and have numerous limitations and caveats. Yet collectively, all 27 studies make a strong, compelling, and surprisingly consistent argument that hippocampal CA1 LTP plays a key causal role in hippocampal learning and memory. The integrative consistency across these 27 different manipulation studies, as well as the fit of the results into known intracellular signaling pathways, justifies the CA1 LTP→Hippocampal Learning hypothesis. We can accept this hypothesis and move on with confidence that the case for causal relevance has been made. What then of the more extended causal hypothesis, that CaMKII→LTP→Learning?

Acknowledging that LTP is a mechanism of learning is not tantamount to demonstrating that CaMKII could only affect Learning by affecting LTP. The reality could just as easily be that CaMKII affects LTP and Learning through non-overlapping channels—that is, LTP←CaMKII→Learning. Determining that a causal factor mediates an effect of an agent on a target—that the factor is part of a mechanism for the target—requires us to be more explicit about the evidential standards for drawing arrows in our causal hypotheses. This requirement leads us to a fourth form of Integration and the topic of the next chapter, Mediation Analysis.

[7]

A DREAM WITHIN REACH: BUILDING AUTOMATED RESEARCH MAPS

1. A MAP OF EXPERIMENTAL RESEARCH

Imagine a glowing map of every phenomenon studied in neuroscience, laid out in constellations of hypothesized causal interactions. Surveying its landscape, we find each tentative causal connection appended with a dependability score, based on the outcomes of the different forms of Integration analyses summarized here. Clicking on any one of these connections, we are linked to a summary of the publications reporting the relevant experiments. We type into the search bar: "highlight all causal paths involving CA1 and CaMKII with dependability scores higher than n" and a legion of phenomena and their connections fade into the background, leaving glowing only the part of the network to which we limited our search. Imagine waking up in the middle of the night with a hunch about CaMKII function and being able to immediately summon this map to explore the implications of your hunch, all based on the published science that has come before.

Absorbing every piece of data ever published on a specific causal hypothesis, sifting stones from gems but discarding nothing, such an interactive map could empower neuroscientists to plan experiments in ways never before possible, to pursue research paths that would otherwise remain hidden. A map such as this could be used to engineer revolutions in neuroscience. We could build this map.

2. LOST IN COMPLEXITY

There is at present a growing consensus among neuroscientists that we must implement better methods for navigating the sea of research publications. We are finite creatures with bounded rationality and limited memory and attention. The published information that can be brought to bear on any one causal hypothesis or on the planning of any single experiment has become too large, too complex, and well beyond the limited capacities of any group of individuals to master. Rather than helping neuroscientists in their quests, the vastness of the published record threatens to drown many of our creative efforts in irrelevance and obsolescence. To tackle this growing problem, we need novel approaches, new ways of working with the published record. We need methods that turn the vastness of the published record away from being a problem and instead make it the tremendous resource it can be.

In contemplating the immensity of the published record, the challenge of organizing *mediating variables* is especially vexing. Whenever we learn that A affects B, our minds reflexively ask how this happens—by what phenomenon C does A affect B ($A{\rightarrow}C{\rightarrow}B$)? Consider the list of an estimated 7000 genes expressed in the brain. Consider the functional states and interactive permutations of the many thousands of proteins that these 7000 genes encode. The synapse alone may include many thousands of different interactions among its hundreds of different proteins (Grant et al., 2005)!

Next consider the cellular processes all of these proteins regulate, the connection patterns of the cells involved, their organization into microcircuits, networks, and large ensembles that must all function together dynamically during the allocation, acquisition, consolidation, reconsolidation, and retrieval of information. How many interactions do these phenomena enter into to mediate learning and memory? It boggles the mind! Unfortunately, in the real world planning of specific experiments and interpreting their results, neuroscientists cannot avoid *ignoring* much of this fast-growing complexity. Otherwise specific experiments wouldn't get done.

Buried in the vastness of the published record, there are undoubtedly troves of unnoticed causal connections and novel hypotheses waiting to be mined by someone, *or something*, with the wherewithal to connect the dots. Because we have yet to discover a way to successfully organize and navigate the immensity of the experimental record—the PUBMED resource alone now includes more than 20 million articles—we mostly (have to) ignore it, and focus instead on tiny pockets of it, cherry-picked for us by our mentors and colleagues, our hunches, or our idle curiosity. Guided by our intuition and no small measure of luck, we can all name instances when, despite all of this complexity, we were able to stumble across a novel causal hypothesis or an experiment that changed the course of our research. But it would be preferable if these occurrences were not so sporadic. There will always be a place in science for lucky accidents and intuition, but neuroscientists need *systematic* ways to connect the dots hidden in the vastness of the experimental record. The prospect of developing such systems draws our attention to a form of Integration essential to the project of deriving models of neural mechanisms from maps of experimental research—that is,

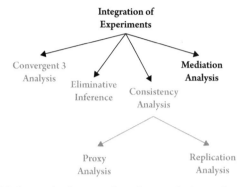

Figure 7.1 Mediation Analysis involves the search for evidence concerning mediating variables to explain *how* an agent phenomenon (A) affects a target (B). As emphasized in the next section, Multi-Connection Experiments are particularly important to this endeavor. Multi-Connection Experiments combine the different kinds of manipulation that occur in Single Connection Experiments (e.g., for a $A{\rightarrow}C{\rightarrow}B$ causal hypothesis, a Positive Manipulation of *A* simultaneously with a Negative Manipulation of *C*, while measuring for *B*, would inform on whether *C* is required for the effects of *A* on *B*).

to Integration by Mediation Analysis. (*See* Fig. 7.1) We turn now to this form.

3. ALIGNING THE ARROWS

Neuroscientists often draw cartoons to summarize informa-tion in research papers and reviews (e.g., diagram in Fig. 6.2). However, it is too easy simply to take such cartoons at face value. What do all of those lines and arrows really represent? What does the placement of the different proteins into illustrated sequences imply about what we should find in the experimental record? How do we justify those arrows? To address these questions rig-orously, we need the Integration methods we already discussed, and we also need additional principles for inferring *mediating causes* (the C in an $A{\rightarrow}C{\rightarrow}B$ causal path). Principles for inferring mediating causes are now the focus of a field of statistical machine learning that utilizes *graphical causal models*, or what we will simply call causal graphs, to represent hypotheses concerning causal connections.

Before we introduce some resources from this field, we wish to be clear on our goals. Causal graphs are a representational tool, a way to represent information. We wish to show how this tool can be used to represent experimental results usefully and compactly, and then how representations of causal processes can subsequently be derived. All of this constitutes first steps toward the glowing map we imagined at the beginning of this chapter.

Two groups, one at UCLA led by Judea Pearl, and one at Carnegie Mellon University led by Clark Glymour, developed the theory of causal graphs using causal diagrams to represent conditional independence relations (Pearl, 2000; Spirtes, Glymour, and Scheines, 2000). One of their many ideas was that causal paths like $A{\rightarrow}C{\rightarrow}B$ can be used to encode the statement that phenomenon B is *independent* of A once the state of C is held fixed or "frozen"—the claim that once C's occurrence is held frozen, variations in A will fail to affect B. For example, translating our CaMKII example into a statement about probabilities, we can use the notation "CaMKII activation→LTP induction→Learning" to represent that the probability that *learning* is conditionally independent of the probability of *CaMKII activation* given *LTP induction*.

Distinct causal graphs often motivate distinct experiments. If we are unsure which of CaMKII→LTP→Learning or LTP←CaMKII→Learning is true, the theory of causal graphs tells us what we can do experimentally to reduce our uncertainty—we can conduct Multi-Connection Experiments. In this type of experiment,

		APS Injection (LTP Fixed)
(CaMKII Varies)	Viral Vector Injection	Group 1 Result: % ± ε
	No Viral Vector Injection	Group 2 Result: % ± ε

Figure 7.2 Assuming that our Negative and Positive Manipulations worked successfully, we take all of the mice who have received AP5 injections and divide that group into those that have received CaMKII viral vector injections (Group 1) and those that have not (Group 2). We represent the results of the hidden platform task for both groups as the mean search time in the target quadrant (%) with an error measure of ε. If the hidden platform tasks for Group 1 do not significantly differ from the results for Group 2, we conclude that the increase in CaMKII levels only affect learning by affecting LTP. In addition to the two groups described in the table, we would also include in the experiment the other groups of mice that never received AP5 injections: mice that received the CaMKII viral vector (Group 4) and those that did not (Group 5). According to previous findings (Poulsonet al., 2007, discussed in Chapter 4 above), hidden platform task results for Group 4 should differ significantly from Group 5.

multiple variables are manipulated at the same time. Although they are not rare, Multi-Connection Experiments are less common in Molecular and Cellular Cognition than the single connection experiments we have talked about so far. The reason is simple: The more complex the experiment, the more things can go wrong and the longer the list of possible confounds.

One possible strategy to distinguish between the CaMKII→LTP→Learning and LTP←CaMKII→Learning models would be to combine a Positive Manipulation of CaMKII with a Negative Manipulation of LTP and then measure learning in a hippocampal task like contextual conditioning or the Morris water maze (*see* Fig. 7.2). To draft our design, recall from Chapter 4 that Poulsen and colleagues used a viral vector to Positively Manipulate CaMKII and get an enhancement in spatial learning on the hidden platform task of the water maze (Poulsen et al., 2007). Suppose that we were to combine the same Positive Manipulation followed by an injection of AP5 to the CA1 region prior to training. AP5 would give us a Negative Manipulation of NMDA receptor activity—activity that is normally required for LTP. If LTP is impaired by the AP5 injections, then we could conclude that the state of LTP had been fixed with this specific Negative Manipulation. If the levels of CaMKII were elevated from the viral vector, that would confirm that CaMKII levels had been Positively Manipulated. Looking at the data from the hidden platform task, we could then ask whether learning was enhanced in the cases where AP5 was administered while CaMKII levels were increased. If learning were unchanged (or even impaired) in the AP5 experimental group despite the enhancement in CaMKII performance, we would have evidence for the CaMKII→LTP→Learning model. On the other hand, if learning were enhanced despite the LTP block with AP5, then the CaMKII→LTP→Learning model would be falsified.

Suppose that learning was enhanced despite the blockage of LTP. Could we then conclude that the model where LTP←CaMKII→Learning is best? Unfortunately, there is a third model that could account for this hypothetical result of our proposed experiment, a model that would have been eliminated if learning didn't vary. (*See* Fig. 7.3.) We would have to design and perform

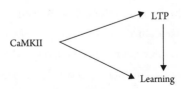

Figure 7.3 A causal graph with a direct connection between CaMKII and Learning could accommodate the hypothetical results of our imagined experiment just as well as LTP←CaMKII→Learning.

additional experiments to resolve the structure of the mechanism CaMKII is affecting.

With this brief thought experiment, we can see the value of Multi-Connection Experiments and their relevance for Mediation Analysis. There are other experimental designs that could be used to help us choose among competing causal models. The relevant experiments might even have been published somewhere already, but lie hidden in some dimly lit corner of the web archives, beyond the reach of our search engines.

Only a generation ago, it was possible for neuroscientists to be familiar with the entire publication record of their field. But this kind of intimacy with the published record is no longer possible. In our age of multidisciplinary studies, often involving traditionally separate fields, neuroscientists are asked to have more than a passing familiarity with neighboring fields. Additionally, the experimental record now grows at a rate that outstrips the human capacity to integrate it. Consequently, we must confront the record with more than personal determination—we must confront it with new technology.

4. CAPTURING THE EXPERIMENTAL LANDSCAPE

The first step toward performing large-scale Mediation Analysis of the type we touched upon in the previous section is to develop an information infrastructure for mapping published experimental reports. Before we infer neural mechanisms and assemble complicated causal networks, we need a workable representation of the available data. We have proposed that the Framework and Integration rules we introduced in earlier chapters be used to develop that representation for Molecular and Cellular Cognition (MCC) research.

The Framework would be used to classify all published MCC experiments, and the Integration tests, such as the Convergent 3, Eliminative Inference, and Consistency Analyses, would be used to identify causal connections and weigh the evidence supporting them (e.g., CaMKII→LTP). Once we have a database of all of the experiments recorded in the field, all causal connections supported by the data, as well as their relative reliability (estimated with the Integration tests described), we can then use Mediation Analysis to determine which overall causal models best fit the constraints provided by that record—we can generate an overall map of the experimental landscape. But we are getting ahead of ourselves. First, it will be useful to develop a simplified representation of all the experiments published in the area that we want to map.

To see how to build a large-scale map representing a collection of experiments—a Network of EXperiments or NEX—it will help to consider how we could build small-scale graphs to represent each experiment individually. The usual (minimal) way to represent an experiment using a causal graph is to include an arrow pointing into a phenomenon to indicate a manipulation, and an arrow leading out of a phenomenon to indicate that a measurement device has detected a response.[1] To keep our examples simple, we will pretend that our target phenomena are our measuring devices. With that idealization in place, we can use a pair of causal graphs to represent some of the 1992 experiments we discussed in detail in earlier chapters, as shown in Figure 7.4.

Contrary to the way that path diagrams may at other times be interpreted, when we use the rules from causal theory, the absence of an arrow between two nodes means that neither phenomenon affects the other directly. Looking at the graphs in Figure 7.4, the absence of an arrow from Knockout to LTP or to Hidden Platform Test means that the knockout only had an effect on these variables

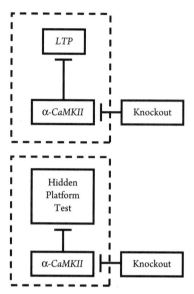

Figure 7.4 Causal graphs representing some of the 1992 experiments. Nodes inside of the dotted-line boxes indicate phenomena found in the system studied (i.e., the animal, including its behavior). Nodes outside indicate iterventions on that system (e.g., a genetic knockout of αCaMKII). We use a flat-headed arrow to represent an inhibitory effect (the outcome being a Target Decrease). Recall that the Hidden Platform Test is a memory test in the Morris water maze, which probes hippocampal-dependent spatial learning. In the Hidden Platform Test, an animal is trained to find a platform submerged under opaque water.

through its effect on αCaMKII—*given the variables in the graph.* This last remark is particularly important to emphasize: It is possible that the knockout procedure directly affected other variables aside from the αCaMKII gene. The omission of these other variables makes these graphs somewhat presumptuous. However, because we are aware of this presumptuousness, we will not let the omission of other variables distract us. We simply keep in mind that these models represent only the information we collected from the specific experiments each represents.

One notable feature of our graphical models is that they can be read more quickly than an article's abstract. If you are somewhat familiar with the phenomena involved, one glance at Figure 7.4 tells you some of the results from the 1992 experiments. These graphs are potentially less ambiguous representations simply because they are less verbose. Will these advantages scale up to representations of collections of experiments—like the collection depicted in Figure 7.5?

Suppose that we take a collection of models, like that illustrated in Figure 7.5, and focus on the overlapping variables (i.e., phenomena) —for example, CaMKII. To represent that CaMKII was studied in each experiment in the collection we're representing, we introduce one node into a Network diagram of Experiments—a NEX—to represent CaMKII (*see* Fig. 7.5). Suppose that in the entire collection of experiments we're representing, some measured the effects of CaMKII manipulation on LTP and others on the hidden platform task. We could then add two additional nodes in our NEX graph, each representing one of these two different overlapping variables, LTP and the hidden platform task (*see* Fig. 7.5). We then draw the appropriate lines from CaMKII to those two variables to represent the experimental results (*see* Fig. 7.5). We will now have represented numerous experiments using only three nodes.

To convey more information about what was learned in these numerous experiments, we could use different kinds of arrowheads to represent the kinds of causal connections that have been discovered, given the experimental evidence thus far. For example, if only Non-Intervention Experiments have been performed and only positive correlations have been found, then we could represent this collection of experiments as "A—B" to indicate that we don't know whether A drives B or B drives A. If we later perform Manipulation Experiments and find that A facilitates B, we could

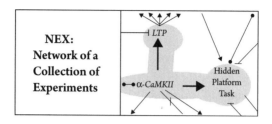

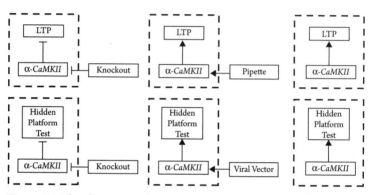

Figure 7.5 The diagram at the top is a region of a NEX (Network of EXperiments) derived from some of the experiments discussed in Chapter 4, embedded within a larger NEX representing other experiments relating those phenomena (CaMKII, LTP, Hidden Platform Task) to other phenomena (not pictured as nodes in the NEX diagram or among the collection of individual experiments below it). The heavily weighted arrows in the NEX indicate that the arrows are supported by all components of the Convergent 3 Heuristic. The pointed tips of the arrows (vs. flat heads) indicate that the relationship between the variables is facilitating instead of inhibitory. Edges that end in dots indicate that an inhibitory relation was found. Edges with a line through them indicate that an experiment was performed but no effect was found (e.g., Null Correlation). The NEX reduces a collection of many small graphs depicting specific published experiments, like the collection depicted in the bottom diagrams of the Figure (and discussed in earlier chapters), to a region in one big graph, enabling us to more quickly survey the published experimental record.

transform that link to $A{\rightarrow}B$. Different arrowheads could be used to distinguish facilitating from inhibitory causal relationships, and the nodes in the network could be used to represent measured phenomena. Finally, experiments involving more than one manipulation or measurement (i.e., Multi-Connection Experiments) could be represented by another convention, such as shading the collection of variables involved (*see* Fig. 7.5).

Representing published information in this way, as a NEX, would provide us with a useful summary of what we think was accomplished in each published experiment, enabling a neuroscientist to very quickly survey the contents of a large number of experimental reports. However, a NEX does not represent neural mechanisms, as that would require the arrows in the NEX to represent transitive causal relationships (e.g., that A causes C by causing B, $A{\rightarrow}B{\rightarrow}C$). But that is not what a NEX represents. Its arrows are simply combinative representations of the results of the specific experiments represented.

Of course, the NEX in Figure 7.5 concerns only a small number of overlapping variables, leaving us to wonder what would happen to the tidiness of such representations as the number of overlapping variables expands. In theory, the density of the network— how much it resembles an unmanageable "hairball"—could be controlled by allowing users to view only the types of connections they wish to examine. For example, users may choose to view only connections that have satisfied all of the Convergent 3 components, or connections that are only weakly supported by the represented experimental reports, or connections involving one or more specific phenomena, and so on. Like an interactive geographical map, the network could be viewed at various grains of detail and landmarks of interest. Thus, a NEX could be used, for example, to survey areas of expected intense research investment and to identify where critical gaps exist and needed resolutions are pressing in the experimental record. In essence, NEXes could be used as explicit representational tools for helping researchers to determine more efficiently where to direct their research efforts, according to their interests and experimental capabilities, and based on findings already reported in the published experimental record.

5. FROM GRAPHS OF EXPERIMENTS TO GRAPHS OF MECHANISMS

A representation of an experimental record (a NEX, like that depicted in Fig. 7.5 above) is not a representation of an assembled neural mechanism. In Chapter 6, we looked at a path diagram—a causal model—that helped make sense of the learning and memory enhancements in 27 different knockout and transgenic experiments (Fig. 6.2). That diagram was a representation of neural mechanisms associated with synaptic plasticity, as opposed to a diagram of an experimental record. The same data required to map an experimental record can also be used to estimate causal models of mechanisms studied in that record, but the two projects should not be confused.

To derive informative, large-scale causal networks representing the structure of neural mechanisms, one might speculate that it could suffice to combine the presumptuous causal models (NEXes) for the mechanisms' hypothesized components. A collection of causal graphs representing the outcomes of distinct experiments could be used to construct a super-graph of the causal system under investigation (Tillman, Danks, and Glymour, 2009). If the variables in a collection of causal graphs overlap (e.g., as $A \rightarrow C \rightarrow B$ and $C \rightarrow D \rightarrow E$ overlap at C) the graphs are in principle combinable. However we must be cautious in how we interpret such graphs, to understand the language in which they are written. For example, recall that the absence of an arrow/edge between two variables, A and B, in a causal graph means that there is no direct causal relationship between the two variables. We could create a hybrid system that merges the functions of a NEX (to represent experiments) with path diagrams (to represent causal structures), to create a NEXpath. In a NEXpath, phenomena would be arranged according to patterns of conditional independence, and each arrow would be indexed to the studies that justify it, just as in a NEX. Noting these similarities, NEXes and NEXpaths must not be confused.

A NEX is a graphical representation of a specific set of experiments (e.g., all published molecular and cellular cognition experiments). By itself, such a graphical representation of experiments does not yield explanations of phenomena of interest, such as memory, attention, desire, emotion, consciousness, and other psychological phenomena. To extract interpretations from such a network, one must use additional strategies that would transform the experimental studies indexed by a NEX into causal paths. Consider the following example of a NEX graph with 15 connections among its variables, omitting for the moment annotations for the considerable experimental evidence behind each of these components. (*See* Fig. 7.6.)

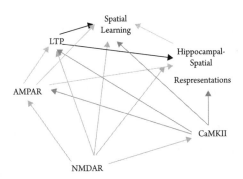

Figure 7.6 A NEX of 15 facilitating connections representing a large collection of experiments.

Based on the causal information represented in the corresponding studies, it might hypothetically be possible to reduce those 15 connections in the NEX into the following causal path:

NMDA receptor $\rightarrow$ CaMKII $\rightarrow$ AMPA receptor $\rightarrow$ LTP $\rightarrow$ Spatial Representations $\rightarrow$ Spatial Learning.

Unlike the 15 connections depicted in the NEX in Fig. 7.6 this causal path has only 5 connections. This is a considerable simplification that would have a significant impact on how such a network could be used to interpret available results and plan future experiments. However, this reduction would also require a great deal of information to be present in the experimental record, as there are typically many causal models that can accommodate a collection of experimental results.

Given a collection of causal models that fit a corpus of experimental results, we imagine that it may be possible to develop "NEXpath scores," quantitative strategies to estimate the impact of specific experiments on our uncertainty. For example, we could track Multi-Connection Experiments that resolve uncertainties in the network's structure (e.g., whenever problems like LTP$\leftarrow$ CaMKII$\rightarrow$Learning vs. CaMKII$\rightarrow$LTP$\rightarrow$Learning are solved). We could also track Identity Experiments that introduced new phenomena out of which a cluster of Connection Experiments grew.

Besides being useful for determining the impact of past experiments on a field of research, NEXpath scores could also be used to estimate the impact of alternative future experimental outcomes. The clarity derived from NEX and NEXpath graphical representations would be a fertile substrate for scientific creativity and intuition. Just as statistical analysis packages have become essential in the analysis of complex experimental data sets, NEXes and NEXpaths could emerge as critical tools in planning future experiments within the complexity of published research.

Of course, assembling a NEX and a NEXpath for all of current neuroscience would involve considerable economic and human resources. It would be more immediately feasible to focus on targeted areas in neuroscience, like molecular and cellular cognition of memory, for example. Although the resulting NEXes would be more limited in their usefulness, such specialized efforts may allow us to develop the many tools we would need for a more global effort. If such a system were to be constructed for the molecular and cellular cognition of memory, how would that affect the direction of future research in this area? Would these tools make us less susceptible to overlooking vital evidence? Would they help us prioritize some experiments over others, and therefore result in scientific acceleration? We do not have definitive answers to these questions, but we have a realistic hope that developments like these will help neuroscientists navigate and effectively take advantage of the growing size of the published experimental corpus, in a fashion that current resources, such as review essays, *never* could. The size of the complete published corpus for even individual causal paths is now just too massive for those old ways. NEXes, and NEXpaths provide a promising set of resources for addressing this problem.

6. NEUROSCIENCE MODELS AND RESEARCH MAPS

Consider in light of this promise the Human Brain Project, an ambitious European modeling project led by Henry Markram that intends to simulate in a supercomputer nothing less than the entire human brain. The impressive and awe-inspiring goal of this initiative follows closely on the footsteps of an earlier initiative, the Blue Brain Project, so named in reference to the Blue Gene supercomputer running

Michael Hines's NEURON software. The Human Brain Project is a vast collaborative initiative involving nearly 100 European institutions, is planned to last ten years (to 2023), and is estimated to cost a whopping 1.19 billion euros. The project is more than just a mega-modeling effort; it is also a strategy to drive future research using modeling resources developed through this impressive effort. In many respects the goals of this unprecedented project are aligned to many of the themes covered in this book, specifically the urgent and immediate need to develop tools that integrate research findings and help neuroscientists plan future experiments. The megamodel projected for the Human Brain Project, if successful, will integrate neuroscience research and result in a virtual platform that will allow scientists to carry out experiments in silico before actually running them in their own laboratories.

Despite its enormous potential and promise, models such as the one proposed by the Human Brain Project may eventually share some of the same complexity problems that burden current literature databases. Among the vast complexity of molecular mechanisms, cell types, circuits, cell ensembles and behavioral phenomena, individual neuroscientists must find their own research tracks. Ultimately, neuroscientists still need to ask the age-old questions that have always guided scientific research: what is known about the phenomena that I want to understand? How reliable is this knowledge? How could I best contribute further understanding? Is it worth pursuing one particular research direction? Why or why not? Without something like the new research tools we're sketching, the unfathomable complexity of the published experimental record could simply be carried over into endeavors like the Human Brain Project. We propose that there is a natural synergy between the research maps we're groping toward and large-scale neuroscience modeling efforts such as the Human Brain Project. We can imagine neuroscientists going back and forth between these two tools: finding direction from research maps and testing ideas in silico, as a means to evaluate the potential impact of their research projects.

7. A MEANINGFUL SEARCH

For the most part, current queries into databases of neuroscience publications are key word searches. You cannot ask an existing search engine whether deficits in LTP cause learning deficits and expect a piece of software to think it through and generate an answer. Rather, you will get a return for linked documents with instances of the terms in your search string. It will then be up to you to go looking for answers to your specific question.

Although keyword search methods represent a vast leap beyond the Kafkaesque chaos of old school archival research, the next leap may span a comparable distance. The next generation of search engines likely will be driven by database designs that resemble our understanding of the knowledge domain they are meant to model. Rather than typing queries like "LTP+Memory+mouse," we will ask, "Does spatial memory in a mouse depend on CA1 LTP?" The computer will look for dependable causal paths with "spatial memory" and "CA1 LTP," and rather than returning a batch of abstracts, we will receive estimated answers to our questions indexed to a summary of the evidence on which the answers were based. Even better, when insufficient evidence is available to answer our questions confidently, our new search systems will tell us what pieces of evidence are missing. Through innovations such as these, experimentalists will be better positioned to perform experiments with a high expected impact on their field. This isn't science fiction. Resources for moving us into the future have already been implemented. We propose that the NEX and Nexpath tools introduced here are a first step toward the development of these search engines.

There are key resources already in place that will be essential for the development of NEXes and NEXpaths. For example, to ensure that there is a common, machine-readable language for communicating data and analyses in neuroscience, the Neuroscience Information Framework (NIF) has developed and maintains a controlled vocabulary, the NIF standard ontology (Larson and Martone, 2009). An "ontology" here is a collection of terms used to model knowledge in some specific domain of understanding. For example, our knowledge that a pyramidal cell is a kind of cell would be documented in a neuroscience ontology by including a term for pyramidal cell, a term for cell, and a relation indicating that one is a subclass of the other. Under the leadership of Maryanne Martone, an accomplished neuroanatomist, the NIF has annotated a massive storehouse of data and developed a search engine that provides neuroscientists with a one-stop shop for online research.

Of course, collecting and organizing data will be just as vital to S2 as the proper storage and retrieval of it. In developing tools for documenting the provenance of neuroscience data—that is, the processes by which neuroscience data is generated—Gully Burns at USC's Information Sciences Institute is leading the way. Burns' tools are based on a framework called KEfED—an acronym for "knowledge engineering from experimental design" (pronounced KAY-fed). In its current implementation, KEfED is part of the BioScholar software package, a system that will enable scientists to document the design of their experiments (e.g., anterograde tract tracing) as well as the measurements and results of that experiment (Russ et al., 2011). Having used KEfED to enter experimental data into a knowledge base, reasoning can then be performed to derive, for example, the pattern and strength of anatomical connectivity

into and out of a collection of brain structures, such as the components of the hippocampal formation. In principle, KEfED could be
used to harvest the kind of data required to build NEXes of collections of experiments and NEXpaths derived from them, as we've
described above.

Finally, knowledge bases in bioinformatics are essentially existence proofs that an experimental record can be encoded to facili-
tate experiment planning and discovery. For example, Ingenuity
Systems has developed a knowledge base that stores information
on genes, proteins, cells, drugs, diseases, and biological pathways
(Sanderson, 2011). The content of the Ingenuity Knowledge Base
can be navigated graphically and used for modeling, prediction, and
experiment planning in conjunction with other Ingenuity research
tools. Although Ingenuity does not use a comprehensive taxonomy
of experiments to structure data, the strides it has made in developing the Ingenuity Knowledge Base are an existence proof for the
literature mapping technology we envision.

8. BEFORE THE FUTURE ARRIVES

Although the technologies we envision are incredibly promising, they will take time to mature to the point we're imagining. So,
what resources do we have for planning neuroscience experiments
today? In the next chapter we will outline a method for research
planning that takes advantage of the Framework and Integration
approaches introduced in earlier chapters, whose actual implementation requires nothing more than some persistence and attention
to detail.

[8]

ARCHITECTURE FOR
EXPERIMENTALISTS

1. LOEWI'S DREAM

Otto Loewi was famous for discovering that acetylcholine mediates communication between nerve fibers and the smooth muscle cells of the heart. At the time of Loewi's experiments, no one was sure whether neurons used electrical sparks to communicate with each other or if there was instead a chemical soup—a neurotransmitter—carrying the message. The experiments that led Loewi to his discovery came to him in a dream, a dream that helped him win a Nobel Prize in 1936. If only we could all have dreams as rewarding as Loewi's! But that seems an unreliable source to count on for fruitful experiment planning. For better or worse, experiment planning is a process we mostly undertake during waking hours.

Relevance, reliability, and decisiveness are among the attributes that we look for in our designs, but no formula readily yields a method that we can expect to satisfy these desiderata. Although we can plan experiments that are interesting because of their design, we cannot guarantee that they will be interesting because of their results. The problem of determining how to choose the next experiment consequently levitates just beyond our grasp. Its solution seems just as ineffable as capturing the force behind an artist's creativity.

Or so one might think. We have already discussed in the previous chapter the power and potential of deriving maps of experiments. In this chapter we will see that the Framework and Integration approaches introduced here afford several additional resources for helping us decide which experiments should be performed next. Although no tool can guarantee ground-breaking results for all, we can offer practical guidelines for identifying experiments that would address identifiable weaknesses and provide missing evidence in an area of interest. These guidelines are grounded in the resources we have introduced so far. As we mentioned before, the Framework and Integration approaches introduced reflect implicit and explicit practices in neuroscience. We have not invented any of the principles we will outline. We have simply organized them into an explicit system.

To make our recommendations concrete, we will work with a live research project in molecular and cellular cognition. We will use a problem we are currently struggling with, an area that is novel and where standard practices and approaches are still mostly missing. Actually, while writing this chapter in early 2010 we worked through some of the challenges to experiment planning that this new research presents. Our chosen topic is memory allocation: the problem of understanding the mechanisms that determine which cells in a circuit are recruited to store a given memory (Silva et al., 2009). As we will see, the Framework and Integration approaches introduced here helped us get clarity concerning the allocation experiments previously carried out as well as in our efforts to identify critical future experiments in this new area of memory research. Once again we acknowledge that undoubtedly there are more deserving topics that we could have used: We simply used one with which we are very familiar to illustrate the concepts we would like to put across in this chapter.

For the discussion in this chapter, we encourage the reader to perform an intellectual exercise. Consider it a challenge. At the time of this writing three research papers have been published on the topic of memory allocation: Han et al. (2007), Han et al. (2009), and Zhou et al. (2009). We will review the experiments reported in those papers, use the S2 Framework to map the results, and plan future experiments. However, before we provide this review, we ask the reader to stop reading this book, study those three papers, and propose critical follow-up experiments for evaluating the central hypothesis and furthering our understanding of memory allocation. Having completed that exercise, we'll then invite the reader to follow our description of the published experiments and our explicit S2 rationale for future experiments to perform. There is no better way to judge the merits of this approach than by actually taking it for a test drive!

2. IN THE DRAFTING ROOM

Before building a structure it is best to draft blueprints, and before drafting blueprints, it helps to assess the needs that the finished structure will meet. Our need is to design experiments that maximize informational returns, supplying us with results that are both relevant to our interests, in terms of testing existing causal hypotheses, and reliable, as assessed across the various methods of Integration we've discussed in earlier chapters. Sometimes you can wing it and a glorious experimental design falls into your lap, as with Loewi and his famous dream. Science at its heart is a game of chance, after all, and the law of large numbers can comfort risk-takers. However, even when you're playing games of chance, there are sometimes ways to lessen your reliance on Lady Luck.

Every experiment-planning problem begins in the midst of some published body of results. This is the backdrop against which the drama of future experiments unfolds, the leverage you have available to bet on future experiments. The planning problem we discuss in this chapter grows out of findings from the 1960s when it was discovered that long-term memory, but not short-term memory, depends on the synthesis of new proteins in the brain (Flexner et al., 1963). Although it was not known what new proteins would be required, over time it became clearer that the most likely suspects would be proteins required for maintaining LTP. Surprisingly, CaMKII turned out to be less important for LTP maintenance than LTP induction and more important for short-term memory than long. By 1994, Bourtchouladze and colleagues in the Silva lab had shown that a transcription factor, cAMP response element-binding protein, or CREB, was critical for LTP maintenance and long-term memory but not for LTP induction or short-term memory (Bourtchuladze et al., 1994). Being a transcription factor, CREB could bind to DNA in a neuron's nucleus and control the transcription of genes into RNA.

Later experiments, conducted by Abel and Bourtchuladze in Kandel's lab showed that a different kinase, protein kinase A (PKA), was also necessary for maintaining CA1 LTP and for normal long-term memory performance in contextual conditioning (Abel et al., 1997). PKA phosphorylates and activates CREB. Therefore, the fact that later phases of LTP and memory depend on these two molecules made sense. CREB could regulate gene transcription, and thereby affect protein synthesis, whereas PKA could induce CREB to do its job.

In the same year that Bourtchouladze published her results on CREB, studies from Tully's laboratory also showed that although lower levels of CREB activity lead to memory deficits in flies (Negative Manipulation), increasing CREB levels (Positive

Manipulation) yields stronger memory (Yin et al., 1994). These findings, along with pioneering Negative Manipulation studies with *Aplysia* (a sea snail) by Pramod K. Dash in Kandel's laboratory, motivated a flurry of research on the role of CREB in memory (Dash, Hochner, and Kandel, 1990). CREB appeared to be part of a memory mechanism conserved across species as diverse as insects, gastropods, and mammals. Over time and much research, evidence was accumulated for a qualitative model to describe that mechanism.

According to the model, postsynaptic activity sufficient to induce long-lasting LTP causes a rise in intracellular cyclic adenosine monophosphate (cAMP) molecules. Increased numbers of cAMP molecules bind to regulatory subunits of PKA molecules. This binding frees catalytic PKA subunits to move into the neuron's nucleus, where they phosphorylate and therefore activate CREB. Once activated, CREB helps to turn on the expression of genes necessary to trigger the late phase of LTP and memory. (*See* Fig. 8.1.)

A few years after the initial CREB findings were first reported, Sheena Josselyn in Mike Davis's laboratory used viral vectors to show that overexpression of CREB in the amygdala—a Positive Manipulation of CREB—was sufficient to enhance emotional memory in rats (Josselyn et al., 2001). More precisely, rats with enhanced CREB levels induced by the inserted viral vector showed superior memory for fear conditioning.[1] Bourtchouladze's Negative Manipulation had been complemented with a fascinating Positive Manipulation of the same phenomena. But there were some wrinkles still to be ironed out.

It turns out that the virus Josselyn used to increase the levels of CREB in the amygdala infected only about 15% of the cells in this structure, leaving the vast majority of amygdala neurons untouched by the Positive CREB Manipulation. Previous electrophysiological

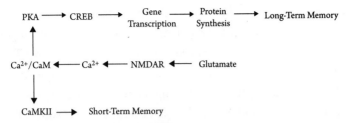

Figure 8.1 PKA is indirectly activated by calmodulin loaded with calcium. When NMDA receptors are activated by glutamate, calmodulin (CaM) is loaded with calcium (Ca/CaM). What is not shown in the graph is that Ca/CaM activates another enzyme (adenylate cyclase) that synthesizes cAMP. cAMP then activates PKA. When PKA is activated, its catalytic subunit moves into the neuron's nucleus to activate CREB, which binds to special sites on DNA (called CRE sites). Once bound, CREB can then regulate the transcription of specific genes into mRNA. Translation of these mRNAs then yields new proteins required for long-term memory.

studies had revealed that a given episode of fear conditioning was known to eventually engage only about one-fourth of the neurons in the amygdala. Assuming that it was activity in the infected neurons that was driving the memory enhancement, how did the fear conditioning memory know to go to the CREB-infected neurons? All things being equal, only a small component of the memory would be expected to end up in the neurons with experimentally manipulated higher CREB activity.

3. THE MEMORY LURE

In a discussion with Silva during a visit to the Davis Laboratory, a potential explanation emerged for Josselyn's findings. Perhaps the higher levels of CREB could be changing amygdala neurons into memory attractors (i.e., they increased the probability that memory was being *allocated* to those neurons). For example, increasing the levels of CREB via the inserted viral vector might increase the levels of sodium channels in amygdala neurons. This increase would make these cells easier to activate and thereby make them ready participants in memory encoding. It was also possible that cells with higher levels of CREB acquired some other new physiological property, making them more likely to encode the fear conditioning memory. Once those neurons were engaged by the conditioning episode, the higher levels of CREB might also raise the odds that the memory for fear conditioning would be consolidated, thus resulting in a memory enhancement compared to mice with normal levels of CREB. A series of new experiments was in order.

At the time of these discussions, the Davis laboratory was about to move from Yale University to Emory University, and Josselyn decided to stay in the Northeast and join the Silva laboratory. After the move, Josselyn reproduced in mice the viral CREB results she had gotten with rats. Once again, she showed that increasing the levels of CREB in approximately 15% of the neurons in the lateral amygdala enhanced fear conditioning performance (Han et al., 2007). To determine whether CREB cells were indeed memory attractors, Josselyn had to show that they were preferentially incorporated into the memory trace encoding the training episode. But, how could one visualize a memory trace? How could one test the CREB →Memory Allocation hypothesis?

The results of Guzowski's work in the laboratories of Barnes and Worley offered a solution (Guzowski et al., 1999). Guzowski had shown that when a hippocampus neuron has recently been active, mRNA for the activity-related cytoskeletal associated protein (ARC) accumulates in its nucleus. With time, the ARC mRNA is carried out of the nucleus for translation into protein. If ARC mRNA is fluorescently labeled, then its expression in the nucleus can be used to identify a cell that is part of that memory's trace, because in tissue slices the nuclei of recently active cells will light up like fireflies against the background of dark inactive cells. Thus, if ARC mRNA fluorescence is found preferentially in the nuclei of CREB enhanced cells during retrieval, this would indicate that increasing CREB levels can bias memory allocation to the cells with the higher levels of this transcription factor. Perhaps, ARC mRNA could be used as a tool to study CREB's role in memory allocation?.

Josselyn used a viral vector to transfect a subset of cells in the lateral amygdala with CREB (Positive Manipulation) and trained the mice in tone conditioning, an amygdala-dependent memory task in which mice learn to respond to a specific tone. After testing the mice for memory retrieval by placing them back in the conditioning chamber and playing the tone used during training, Josselyn found that CREB-enhanced cells (in her CREB Positive Manipulation) were three to four times more likely to show ARC mRNA (i.e., be involved in memory allocation?), indicating recent activity during memory retrieval of tone conditioning. This result was consistent with the CREB allocation hypothesis. In contrast, decreasing the levels of CREB (Negative Manipulation), via a mutant CREB gene that interfered with CREB function, had the opposite effect. Cells transfected with mutant CREB were only one-twelfth as likely to express ARC mRNA. Thus, a Positive Manipulation of CREB in a subset of cells in the lateral amygdala seemed to increase the probability of memory allocation to those cells, whereas a Negative Manipulation of CREB had the opposite effect.

Later on in her own laboratory, Josselyn and her post-doctoral fellow Han also ran several control experiments critical for interpreting the results of the CREB experiments described above (Eliminative Inference). They showed that CREB was needed for the results obtained, because replacing it in the viral vectors with a bacterial protein with no known function in mammals (beta-galactosidase or Lac Z) had no effect on the ARC expression patterns. They also showed that tone conditioning (i.e., learning) was critical for the effects of the CREB Manipulation on ARC mRNA patterns, as omitting conditioning failed to have an appreciable effect on ARC mRNA nuclear patterns. Finally, they showed that changing CREB levels after memory allocation had taken place (i.e., introducing the viral infection after training) had no effect on ARC mRNA nuclear expression patterns. Without these control experiments, it would have been very hard to interpret the Positive and Negative Manipulation Experiments just described. Recall from previous chapters that control experiments of this sort are a crucial component of Integration.

The data from these studies suggested that neurons with the viral-delivered CREB were preferentially active during encoding and retrieval of the tone/shock memory. However interesting, the hypothesis that CREB levels somehow determine which cells in the amygdala store a given memory was far from being proven. For example, it was possible that CREB simply increases the levels of ARC mRNA, and that the cells with nuclear ARC mRNA signals are actually not involved in the tone memory! In other words, Josselyn and colleagues used nuclear ARC mRNA expression as a tool to determine which amygdala cells were involved in tone memory, but unfortunately there were very little data demonstrating that ARC mRNA expression can be used as a tool to study memory allocation. Although this idea is consistent with Guzowski's previous findings, it is unlikely that ARC mRNA expression reflects only a recently active neuron's participation in memory processes. Myriad other stimuli could engender neuronal activity that activates ARC mRNA, and it is possible that some of these other stimuli may be related to CREB function, while being unrelated to memory. Additional Tool Development experiments were needed for studies of memory allocation.

4. HUSHING THE FIREFLIES

To hedge against ARC mRNA artifacts, Yu Zhou and colleagues in the Silva laboratory carried out further Tool Development Experiments to study memory allocation. They devised two alternative and very different strategies to measure memory allocation (Zhou et al., 2009). One way to test for the function of a phenomenon that cannot be measured directly is to see what happens when you eliminate it. If the memory was indeed in the cells with the higher levels of CREB, then silencing those specific cells should cause forgetting. If the memory was not in those cells, then inactivating them during recall should have little or no effect on behavior in the appropriate memory tests.

To reversibly silence the cells infected with the CREB virus, Zhou borrowed a strategy first developed in Ed Callaway's laboratory. Callaway's group had shown that the drosophila gene for the allatostatin receptor could be used to damp down activity in mammalian neurons. Delivering its ligand, the allatostatin peptide, activates the receptor, which in turn activates specific potassium channels, thus inhibiting action potentials (Tan et al., 2006). Zhou and colleagues cloned the drosophila allatostatin receptor into the CREB gene-enhanced virus, so that all cells infected with the viral CREB also expressed the drosophila allatostatin receptor (Zhou et al., 2009). During tone testing following tone-conditioning, the mice transfected with the CREB virus and treated with allatostatin froze much less than similarly transfected mice treated with a control peptide. When the viral CREB mice were later given another recall test, but this time without the allatostatin treatment, they showed normal memory. These results suggest that allatostatin inactivation could be used as a tool to study memory allocation.

The results just described were also complemented with a series of control experiments that tested this new tool and key implications of the CREB→Memory Allocation hypothesis. For example, when CREB-enhanced cells were inactivated during training, and then inactivated again before testing, no amnesia was found. Inactivation during training kept those cells from firing and therefore from participating in the encoding of the memory, despite the inserted CREB transgene. Consequently, inactivating those cells during testing did not cause amnesia because those cells did not encode the memory for tone conditioning. The memory was encoded instead by other cells active during training.

Results from a study led by Han in Josselyn's own lab (now located in Toronto) converged with Zhou's (Han et al., 2009). Rather than silencing the CREB virus cells with the allatostatin system, Han used a diphtheria toxin/genetic strategy to kill those specific neurons. Eliminating the CREB-enhanced neurons after training caused amnesia for tone conditioning, but eliminating a comparable percentage of neurons independent of CREB levels resulted in a much less pronounced memory deficit. Altogether these findings showed that the diphtheria toxin and allatostatin methods could be used as tools to study memory allocation. They also converged with results where ARC mRNA expression was used to study this memory phenomenon.

To further test whether cells with viral CREB were in fact memory trace cells for tone conditioning, Zhou looked at synaptic potentiation (Zhou et al., 2009). Previous data had shown that tone conditioning potentiates synapses between thalamic inputs and lateral amygdala cells and that this potentiation is critical for tone conditioning behavior. In fact, a significant amount of evidence indicates that this potentiation is a key component of the memory trace for tone conditioning (for a review, *see* Sah et al., 2008). Therefore, if a disproportionate amount of the tone conditioning memory is allocated to cells transfected with the CREB virus, after tone conditioning these cells should have higher synaptic strengths than other cells in the lateral amygdala. This meant that synaptic potentiation could potentially be used as yet another tool to study memory allocation.

Indeed, Zhou and colleagues (2009) showed that tone conditioning increased synaptic strength in lateral amygdala neurons and that these increases were higher in the cells transfected with the CREB virus. In contrast, a much smaller potentiation was found in the cells from trained animals that were transfected with a control virus and in other nontransfected lateral amygdala cells. Thus, the impact of a Positive Manipulation of CREB on memory allocation was studied with four very different tools (ARC, allatostatin, diphtheria, potentiation), and the results of all of these experiments were consistent with the CREB→Memory Allocation hypothesis.

The studies of memory allocation described so far were focused on tone conditioning. The amygdala, however, is involved in other forms of memory, including taste aversion, and it would be important to determine whether CREB also affects the allocation of those other memories (another form of Proxy convergence). The gist of conditioned taste aversion is easy to grasp. Animals and people avoid new foods that make them sick. They associate specific flavors and smells in the new food with the malaise that follows, even when the nausea comes long after the consumption of the new food. As they had shown with the tone conditioning experiments, Zhou and colleagues (2009) showed that inactivating the CREB-enhanced cells during recall caused amnesia for conditioned taste aversion! This was yet another independent replication of the effects of a Positive Manipulation of CREB on memory allocation: increasing the levels of CREB in a subset of cells of the lateral amygdala increased the probability that those cells were involved in memory, whether that memory involved tone conditioning or conditioning taste aversion.

5. GETTING EXCITED

The experiments presented in this chapter so far converge on the hypothesis that CREB enhancement affects memory allocation in individual neurons of the lateral amygdala. We saw previously that Mediation Analysis is a compelling strategy to strengthen causal hypotheses. In other words, figuring out how CREB affects memory allocation would strengthen the CREB→Memory Allocation hypothesis. In 2006, Nestler and Malenka's laboratories were studying the role of CREB in the nucleus accumbens in mechanisms of drug addition, and they published results indicating that CREB regulates the transcription of genes involved in modulating a cell's excitability (Dong et al., 2006). If during training some amygdala cells are more excitable than others, those cells will more likely be engaged by the training experience and come to encode the memory. Cell excitability could be a mediating cause of the CREB→Memory Allocation hypothesis.

To test this idea, Zhou and colleagues (2009) decided to determine whether the lateral amygdala cells with viral CREB insertions have higher excitability than other lateral amygdala cells. Because it is very difficult to measure excitability during learning episodes directly, Zhou used indirect methods. Taking tissue slices from mice transfected with the CREB virus and from nontransfected controls, Zhou and collaborators showed that neurons with the viral-encoded CREB do fire action potentials more readily than other lateral amygdala cells. And once these neurons are activated, they also fire more action potentials than do control neurons. Once neurons fire, their membranes become hyperpolarized, so that they resist firing again immediately following activity. The CREB virus-enhanced cells showed this post-action potential hyperpolarization, but it was smaller, suggesting that less stimulation would be needed to make these cells fire again. Hence the *intrinsic* excitability of CREB-enhanced cells was elevated. Even more importantly, Zhou and colleagues showed that the CREB-enhanced lateral amygdala cells needed less synaptic stimulation to fire action potentials than did nontransfected lateral amygdala cells. Cells with elevated CREB thus were shown to have higher *synaptic excitability,* a result consistent with the CREB→Excitability hypothesis.

Excitability was not the only potentially mediating phenomenon to explain CREB's effect on memory allocation in individual neurons. Another hypothesis based on previous findings was that higher levels of CREB might increase the number of synapses ready to undergo potentiation. The synapse hypothesis was plausible, but synaptic measurements in amygdala cells transfected with the CREB virus did not find any evidence for it (Zhou et al., 2009). Thus, in planning which experiments to perform next, we should only choose to investigate the synapse hypothesis of memory allocation if we perceive a flaw in these negative results.

Now that we have a view of the current landscape on this issue of CREB and memory allocation, let's explore the kinds of additional experiments that could be performed next. This is a good place for the reader to try his or her hand at applying the Convergent 3 and other aspects of the S2 taxonomy we've described, to represent graphically what the experiments just described have accomplished and what would be interesting to pursue next.

6. SCHEMATIZING OUR DREAMS

The backdrop is now complete. With a few simplifications, we have reviewed most of what has been done to study memory allocation in amygdala neurons up to 2012. What experiments should be performed next?

Although the number of experiments we have reviewed is small, their complexity makes it a challenge to hold them all in mind at once. To overcome this limitation, we start by recording each experiment using a table—what we will call a NEX Schema. To build a NEX Schema for the allocation experiments, we merely list in the leftmost column all of the *agents* and their *targets* in NEX format, and in the right three columns we check which among the Convergent 3 experiments have been performed. Because so many indirect measures were used to operationalize memory allocation, it is helpful to list those measures separately beneath each causal graph. (*See* Table 8.1.)

Even a casual inspection of this NEX Schema shows that the majority of experiments supporting the CREB→Memory Allocation connection are Positive Manipulations. No Non-Intervention Experiments have been performed, and so far only one Negative Manipulation supports this connection. And that single Negative Manipulation was carried out using just one of the four tools developed in these experiments to measure memory allocation (ARC mRNA patterns). The requirements of a Consistency Analysis include repetition of key experiments with the same and alternative methods. The demands of Eliminative Inference imply that we

Table 8.1 A NEX Schema: A Table Constructed by Hand to Keep Track of Experiments that Have Already been Performed.

	Positive Manipulation	Negative Manipulation	Non-Intervention
CREB→FC allocation (ARC)	Yes	Yes	
CREB→FC allocation (Allatostatin)	Yes		
CREB→CTA allocation (Allatostatin)	Yes		
CREB→FC allocation (potentiation)	Yes		
CREB→FC allocation (diphtheria)	Yes		
CREB→Neuron excitability (intrinsic)	Yes		
CREB→Neuron excitability (synaptic)	Yes		

With the Convergent 3 Heuristic and other Integration methods, this table could help us identify additional experiments that could be performed to strengthen the causal connections explored. FC: Fear conditioning; CTA: conditioned taste aversion. The tags mentioned between brackets in the table refer to methods used for the experiments outlined.

should actively come up with alternative explanations for CREB's role in memory allocation and that we should then systematically address those models.

What kinds of information are we thereby missing by not having done additional experiments suggested by the S2 Framework? We stressed before that Non-Intervention Experiments are critical for determining whether a connection suggested by a manipulation experiment, Positive or Negative, reflects the normal functioning of the system. It is conceivable that although experimentally manipulated changes in CREB can affect memory allocation in individual neurons, CREB may not normally be directly involved in this memory process. Non-Intervention Experiments minimize artificial manipulations and rather are designed to determine whether two phenomena co-vary under nonexperimental conditions. Non-Intervention Experiments relating the phenomena at issue here could test whether lateral amygdala cells allocated to a given memory are more likely to have normally higher CREB levels before training and whether cells that normally have lower CREB levels at time of training are more likely to be excluded from the allocated memory trace.

We also stressed that Negative Manipulation Experiments are critical to establish that a given phenomenon is an essential contributing cause to another phenomenon. Because individual neuron components of allocated memories cannot be measured directly, the three papers we summarized developed four different tools to measure this phenomenon indirectly: ARC mRNA patterns, allatostatin-driven inactivation, diphtheria-driven cell death, and synaptic strength measures. Convergence among the results of the Positive Manipulation Experiments using these four tools increases our confidence in the reality of the results, affording *proxy convergence*—that is, convergence found in a Proxy Analysis. Additionally, the Convergent 3 Analysis suggests that successful Negative Manipulation Experiments demonstrating convergence with the Positive Manipulation results would increase our confidence that CREB is essential for memory allocation in individual amygdala neurons. Even the repetition of identical experiments to the ones already described by other laboratories (Replication Analysis) would also strengthen our confidence in the results outlined.

As we've stressed, working out the mediating causes for a hypothesized causal connection like CREB→Memory Allocation is also an effective strategy to increase the evidence for the strength or reliability of that connection (Mediation Analysis). In an attempt to do exactly that, Zhou and colleagues showed that increases in CREB enhance the excitability of lateral amygdala neurons and that this may explain the molecules' impact on memory allocation. Their work expanded the original CREB→Memory Allocation connection to include excitability: CREB →Excitability→Memory Allocation. We could next draft a separate NEX Schema for this expanded hypothesis to see exactly what kind of evidence has been found for it so far and what kinds of experiments still need to be carried out.

Although she investigated the CREB→Excitability hypothesis, Zhou did not test whether excitability itself is connected to memory allocation in individual neurons (Excitability→Memory Allocation). Thus, it remains possible, in light of all the data presented so far, that memory allocation and excitability are two independent effects of CREB: Excitability←CREB→Memory Allocation. To demonstrate that excitability is connected to memory allocation, we would have to design experiments to test whether increases or decreases in excitability, independent of any changes in CREB, affect memory allocation to any given cell. We would also need to test, prior to training, whether normal variations in the excitability of lateral amygdala neurons are associated with memory allocation. The first experiments would involve Positive and Negative Manipulations, whereas the second would involve Non-Interventions. Again, in this series of experiments, it would help to measure allocation with multiple methods for multiple memory types and determine whether the results are consistent across labs, in the way we suggested above regarding our two modes of Consistency Analyses (Proxy and Replication Analyses, respectively).

We have so far focused on planning around the CREB→Excitability→Allocation causal path. If a compelling connection between excitability and memory allocation emerges out of the experiments just outlined, then one would need to expand this causal path. Because CREB regulates the expression of genes, one possibility would be to test which CREB-dependent genes are responsible for the increase in excitability affecting allocation. Previous studies suggested that a specific sodium channel subunit (Scn1b) could be responsible for this change in excitability (for a review, *see* Silva et al., 2009). Therefore, we could expand the causal path to include this subunit: CREB→Scn1b→Excitability→Allocation. Testing this expanded causal path would include using the Convergent 3 and other Integration tools to test the following three previously untested but potential connections in lateral amygdala neurons: CREB→Scn1b, Scn1b→Excitability, and Scn1b →Allocation.

Parallel to our effort to extend the allocation path in individual neurons downstream of CREB activation—that is, between CREB and allocation—we could also extend this causal path upstream. Previously we mentioned that calcium, coming into the cell through NMDA receptors, could lead to the activation of adenylate cyclase, an enzyme that synthesizes cAMP, a second-messenger signaling molecule. cAMP then activates PKA, and PKA in turn phosphorylates and activates CREB. Activated CREB goes on to stabilize LTP and hence contribute to long-term memory (*see* Fig. 8.1). Could this causal path, NMDA receptor→Adenylate Cyclase→PKA, also be required for CREB's role in memory allocation? If so, we could connect the causal paths leading to CREB in memory consolidation with the paths leading to CREB in memory allocation: NMDA receptor→Adenylate Cyclase →PKA→CREB→Scn1b→Excitability→Allocation. Bridging these two causal paths would allow us to leverage insights into the mechanisms of memory consolidation directly into our efforts to understand those of memory allocation. But how would we test this causal chain?

The obvious answer would be to use the Integration tools we have been discussing so far. Given the evidence we have surveyed in this book, we suspect that the closer to CREB we stay (e.g., by carrying out experiments that test the PKA→memory allocation connection), the less surprising our results will be, and that the further from CREB we move (e.g., by deciding next to test the NMDA receptor→allocation hypothesis), the more risky our next experiments would be (but also potentially more revealing).

7. THE HIDDEN PALACE

Successfully performing any of the experiments just outlined would expand the knowledge acquired in the memory allocation experiments we've surveyed. Which experiment is the best one to perform next is an open question. One way to address it would be to ask which part of the fully Integrated hypothesis, NMDA receptor→Adenylate Cyclase→PKA→CREB →Scn1b→Excitability →Allocation, if confirmed, would produce *the most novelty*? NMDA receptors are quite removed from CREB activity and from memory allocation in individual neurons, and therefore demonstrating experimentally that they are involved in this memory phenomenon, and that their effects involve CREB and excitability, would be a significant step in testing this causal path.

Another way to determine the next best experiment would be to ask what experiment, if successful, would have *the biggest impact* in further securing *the part of the hypothesis that we have already tested*—namely, CREB→Excitability→Allocation. Establishing a mechanism for CREB's role in memory allocation would be important because it would give the CREB→Allocation hypothesis a great deal of credibility. Scientists are understandably wary of venturing too far from a set of findings when the grounds for those findings are still shaky. The lack of an established mechanism for a causal effect makes for very shaky ground indeed. So, perhaps the best next experiment is the one that would cement the mechanistic basis for CREB's role in memory allocation in individual neurons—for example, experiments testing the CREB → Scn1b → Excitability → Allocation part of our fully integrated hypothesized causal path.

Taking an even more conservative approach, perhaps the best next experiments would be those designed *to strengthen evidence for what we have found so far*, before venturing out further. We already saw that most of the experiments supporting the CREB→ Excitability→Allocation hypothesis were Positive Manipulations. This is a potentially dangerous situation because a systematic artifact imbedded in our Positive Manipulations could alter the results in ways that do not reflect normal cellular function. For example, an unknown feature of cells virally transfected with the CREB vector could alter memory allocation in ways unrelated to the normal function of CREB. CREB and memory allocation in individual neurons is a new area of study, and perhaps the most important experiments to do next may be those designed to strengthen the connections for which we already have some evidence. Negative manipulations and Non-Interventions could really strengthen the CREB→Excitability→Allocation hypothesis, in the special ways these types of experiments contribute to completed Convergent 3 cases.

On the other hand, we may be intrigued by the success of the previously surveyed experiments and seek to *extend those findings* by carrying out additional Positive Manipulation tests of the CREB→Allocation hypothesis. Although this option is the least likely to produce novel results, it is often the approach chosen in practice by many labs. We already suggested that very large numbers of repetitions of key experiments may be a considerable problem that contributes to the lack of citations for a great part of the published (and funded!) neuroscience literature. But without a reliable map to help us determine what ground we have already covered and where we need to go, we often cling to familiar paths.

Beyond the duplication experiments just mentioned, any of the other experiments sketched above could be highly informative at this stage of the CREB-memory allocation investigation. We hope that the process of graphing the results that have been obtained so far in this new area illustrates the potential power of the framework and Integration approaches we introduced here. Imagine automating this process, so that we—individual scientists and labs, journal editors and reviewers, funding agencies—could accurately turn thousands of experimental reports into networks of experiments (*see* Chapter 7). Imagine then an automated system that can turn those representations of experiments into the most likely causal paths that integrate those results (NEXpaths representing neural mechanisms; *see* Chapter 7).

Of course, there is no guarantee that in having performed the right experiments at the right time, one's paper will be well received. Aesthetic appreciation for experiments is often a subjective matter and it is hard to imagine ever removing this critical component from science. Unfortunately, at present, virtually the entire process of deciding who gets published in which journal, who gets praise for their work, and who gets the next big grant for a promising series of experiments *is equally subjective*. Through the peer review process we do the best we can, but the lack of expertise required to gage the merits of multidisciplinary work against the entire backdrop of what has been accomplished, our own biases and myopathies, personal relationships across the profession, and reputation (or lack thereof), are well-known worries concerning peer review and all too frequently get in the way of fair reviews. This is another reason why we need some method of objectively assessing the potential contribution of a proposed series of experiments to complement all of the other approaches we use for these purposes. Aesthetic appreciation, our intuitions, and our creativity will always have a key role, but we hope that the clarity afforded by tools such as NEXes and NEXpaths, along with their potential automation in the technology of the here-and-now, will bring some much needed objectivity into the process of evaluating, publishing, and funding science.

The relevance of research findings cannot be accurately gaged solely by their reception in the scientific community. One could conceivably build a palace of exquisite data that goes unnoticed. We have to lament the loss in the deluge of scientific publications, even if rare, of thoughtfully planned and carefully executed experiments that yield novel and ground-breaking results. We all wonder about which features critically distinguish work of potentially high impact from work that is merely highly visible. We hope that these are the kinds of questions that the resources described here—the multiple aspects of Integration, NEXes, and NEXpaths—will help us address in an objective manner. We seek not just to know these answers to satisfy idle curiosity, but more importantly, to do more efficient high-impact science. We wish to develop a science of experiment planning.

[9]

THE FUTURE SCIENCE OF EXPERIMENT PLANNING

1. CHANGING THE WEATHER

Mark Twain is sometimes credited with the saying, "Everybody complains about the weather, but nobody does anything about it" (although Twain may have gotten this quip from Charles Dudley Warner). Rather than focusing on the vexing problems that face science in an age of information overload, our purpose has been to search for solutions. The Framework and Integration approaches we reviewed here systematize concepts of Convergence and Consistency we believe will help bring those solutions. With studies of experimental research underway, the needed data for developing an empirical theory of rational experiment planning will finally become available. How might the search for and development of such a theory proceed? What will be the fundamental questions in such a field?

On our view, the first question we must ask is: "How have researchers in fact been choosing their experiments, up until now?" More specifically, what are the principles, implicit or explicit, used by neuroscientists in determining which experiment to carry out next? A closely related question is, "How do researchers in different fields weight the evidence behind a given hypothesis?" Can these principles be used systematically to determine what is known, and what we are uncertain about? The second question is: "How can we improve the experimental choices that researchers have in fact been making?" Can we develop tools (e.g., maps of published information) to inform these choices? We must be especially cautious when addressing this second question, and not overlook the possibility that the strategies and tools we develop could make our choices worse.

The Framework and Integration approaches discussed here were derived from practices commonly used in molecular and cellular neuroscience. Implicitly or explicitly, the ideas we discussed have already been used for many years to interpret and plan experiments in neuroscience and in other areas of biology that use molecular tools, such as cancer, immunology, developmental biology, and so forth. The general principles of Consistency and Convergence are at the heart of how scientists evaluate results and plan experiments, and these two principles are the basis for the specific Framework and Integration principles articulated in this book. This in fact is one of their main strengths: they are tried and true! Indeed, few molecular and cellular biologists would dispute the usefulness of the Framework and Integration approaches discussed here, and we have simply championed their systematic and explicit use during experiment planning in a specific area of neuroscience (molecular and cellular cognition). We imagine that modified implementations of the general principles of Convergence and Consistency would apply to other fields of neuroscience. More importantly, we proposed taking these approaches from the realm of single experiments and pencil and paper, to the realm of computerized automation, where they could be used to design large-scale maps of experiments.

2. WE ARE RIGHT, BUT JUST IN CASE . . .

Despite our enthusiasm for the Framework and Integration approaches discussed here, and despite the many arguments, case studies, and examples that illustrate their application and value, we cannot and should not ignore the possibility that the tools and approaches we are championing could make matters worse. Could we develop strategies to objectively test some or all of the ideas proposed here? For example, the Convergent 3 is central to many of the ideas presented here. Could we devise strategies to determine whether results that survive the scrutiny of a Convergent 3 Analysis are more reliable and/or have a bigger impact than results that do not? What about results that are supported by Consistency, Eliminative Inference, or Mediation Analyses? Are they too more likely to be more reliable and therefore have a more lasting and bigger impact than results that do not?

Tools for citation analysis are among the most obvious candidates for addressing this type of question. For example, if the ideas presented here have merit, then we would expect that in general research papers that are consistent with the ideas articulated here (e.g., adhere to the Convergent 3) would be cited more often than those that do not. Scientists cite other work in their own publications to give credit for important findings and ideas, provide background and context for their own research projects, and lend credibility to their own results. If the members of a scientific community are the best judges of the quality of work in their field— a not implausible assumption—then citation numbers might be expected to reliably indicate some measure of research impact and quality. We might expect that in general (ignoring those diamonds in the rough) most work receiving few or no citations has been judged by the broader community to be either irrelevant or unreliable. Of course, we should not confuse such judgments with reality. Sometimes the Fates work against an article receiving the attention it is due. Nevertheless, it stands to reason that tools designed for the quantitative study of citation patterns in science—that is, scientometrics—should prove useful for addressing descriptive questions in efforts to test the merits of the ideas presented in this book.

On the other hand, and to the best of our knowledge, no tools currently exist for directly addressing questions concerning how to best improve experiment planning and interpretation. We will therefore have to invent such tools. Perhaps in the future, tools such as NEXes and NEXpaths (Chapter 7) will enable us to develop models for predicting the effects of proposed experiments based on published findings in neuroscience—and perhaps in other disciplines, too. These developed models could be tested against the results of experiments as they are published and disseminated. The most reliable of such models could become valuable tools for guiding experimenters down research paths and to maximize the relevance and reliability of their work.

3. GLAMOUR OR PRESTIGE?

Citation measures offer a promising initial basis to design tools to answer descriptive questions about experiment choice. But citation measures have important, well-known shortcomings. First, work is sometimes highly cited because it receives extensive and sustained criticism. A now infamous paper on cold fusion, written by Fleischmann and Pons (1989), has been cited nearly 900 times (ISI Web of Knowledge, 4/26/13). Most of those citations are likely criticisms, given that the paper has become a case study in controvertial science. Sometimes high citation numbers do not reflect high scientific regard, but perhaps these cases are outliers.

A second weakness worth explicit mention is that citation numbers offer only a very indirect and relative scale for assessing science quality and impact. In most cases, the number of citations one can expect depends on the size of the research community, and the publication frequency of that community. Some communities, for example, might publish larger numbers of relatively smaller experimental projects. Publications in areas of science where fewer people work obviously can be expected to receive fewer citations.

A third weakness is that citation numbers can be driven by a lab's size and research productivity, rather than the quality of its work. Larger labs pump out more students and post-docs, who in turn cite the work of their former lab mates. This is not merely self-promotion. Many students and post-docs take their mentors' and former colleagues' work as their own starting points, and that is grounds for citation. The quality of highly cited work can thereby be confounded by research and training lineages.

The last weakness we will mention concerns the disparity between information sharing and consumption. There is no guarantee that a paper being cited is actually being read (Frey and Rost, 2008). Sometimes papers will be cited because others have cited them previously, because it's expected, because one doesn't wish to offend a colleague, or simply because the published and indexed abstract looks relevant to the authors' work. In these cases, citation numbers fail to track a process of critical evaluation and real use (Simkin and Roychowdhury, 2005; 2007).

Clearly, many warranted complaints have been leveled at the use of citation numbers as measures of a paper's quality and impact. However, judging by their wide use, it is also clear that scientists do not think that citation numbers are a useless measure. Perhaps the most reasonable hypothesis is that citation is just a noisy measure, and that we must be careful in the ways we describe it and the conclusions we draw from it. This makes citation measures little different from many other tools we routinely count on to get jobs done. Simply put, we don't know the value of citation numbers as a predictor of research quality because we haven't run any of the appropriate tests. To leverage citation as a quality indicator, we will therefore need to validate it, taking into consideration all of the potential pitfalls and seeing whether the signal beats out the noise.

4. BRACING FOR IMPACT

Let's start with consensus. Every scientist knows that citations matter because publications matter. Citation measures—such as *impact factor*—are used to gage a journal's prominence in its research community. They are in turn used to calculate the relative contributions of individual scientists to their field—for example, the *h-factor*. They are also used to estimate the intellectual influence that an individual paper has on a research community.

Eugene Garfield, the founder of the Institute for Scientific Information (ISI), popularized many of the citation measures used today. Garfield helped to establish the citation index for academic papers that is now a component of the ISI Web of Knowledge (owned presently by Thomson Scientific). For each paper documented in the Web of Knowledge, there is a corresponding list of the articles cited in it, and later articles that cite it.

To believe that any connection exists between citation numbers and the relative importance of scientific studies, we must make at least two substantive—albeit familiar—assumptions. First, we must assume that scientists will typically cite work that they deem *reliable*. If scientists cite papers for the sake of criticism just as often as for support, then any citation measure will be useless for gaging judgments of quality. Second, we must assume that papers are cited because they are deemed *relevant* to the solution of a specific research problem. It is not enough that an experimental result be regarded as good science. The result must also make a contribution to a specific research topic. If we accept these two assumptions, then we have reason to calculate scientometrics.

One sign of the high quality of a study might be its publication in a high-impact journal. Similarly, the quality of a particular scientist's career might be gaged by his or her h-index. The h-index provides a measure that balances the impact of a researcher's work against publication productivity. It is calculated by sorting a researcher's papers, from the highest cited to the lowest cited, numbering them from 1 to n. The calculator then proceeds down the list to find the first paper whose list number is equal to or less than its citation number. For example, at the end of 2010, Nobel laureate Eric Kandel had an h-index of 141, meaning that he had 141 articles that had been cited 141 or more times (ISI Web of Knowledge, queried 04/26/13).

These and other scientometrics measures reflect the raw number of paper citations and so contain no more information than is contained in that record. We cannot look at Kandel's h-index and see, for example, the instrumental role he played in articulating the molecular mechanisms of learning. We cannot look at the *Annual Review of Neuroscience*'s high impact factor and determine the extent to which its review papers have guided new experimentation in neuroscience.

Impact factor measures alone also fail to answer a question we've pressed numerous times throughout this book. Although the

Annual Review of Neuroscience has a high impact factor score, it has also published papers that have hardly been cited (i.e., <4 citations), despite the fact that some of these papers were published more than 20 years ago. Similarly, between 1981 and 2001, the *Journal of Neuroscience*, which publishes mainly primary research articles, published more than 1,000 papers that have received fewer than 10 citations. Over the same time period, and in that same journal, more than 1,000 papers have received 195 citations or more. Why did some publications in this high-impact journal receive fewer than 10 citations, whereas others received close to 200? Does this purely numerical difference indicate any measure of a paper's reliability, novelty, and relevance? Answers to these questions backed by more than mere intuition could be a great aid toward increasing science's efficiency.

Finally, consider the impact factors of the journals themselves. Less than 50% of neuroscience journals have an impact factor greater than 3. But the five journals with the highest impact factors all have scores greater than 14. Is it the quality of the papers published in these five journals that drives these differences? Is it the reputations of the scientists and labs publishing there? What exactly do these numerical differences mean? Should these scores matter at all to an objective evaluation of research quality and impact on the field? We might be able to answer these questions if we had metrics for a paper's relevance and reliability.

5. IS CONVERGENCE ALCHEMY?

Suppose that we constructed a citation analysis focused solely on primary experimental reports. We could narrow our analysis further by focusing only on papers reporting on Connection Experiments, thereby setting aside papers that report on new tools, descriptions of phenomena, review papers, opinion papers, and the rest. We could further narrow our analysis by choosing a specific research topic in a specific field, recognized as such by a community of scientists. For example, we could collect a sample of papers from PubMed by searching for "LTP and Memory," which as of April 2013 returned a list of 2595 papers. Given that it takes time for researchers to become aware of recent publications and cite them, we will have to control for the date of publication. We could do this by sorting papers according to their year of publication.

The remaining sample could then be submitted to an analysis where for each paper we detail the total list of causal connections investigated and the main hypotheses tested. For each hypothesis investigated, we could construct a checklist of the different kinds of Connection Experiments in the study, according to the components of the Framework discussed—namely, Negative Manipulations, Positive Manipulations, and Non-Interventions. Having compiled our data on each paper, we could then ask whether there is a correlation between citation measures for the paper and the extent to which it conformed to the Integration principles discussed here.

As an example, consider a paper published by Karl Giese and colleagues in 1998, a paper whose results we briefly mentioned in Chapter 6. Having carried out a Convergent 3 analysis of the contents of that paper, we see that only Negative Manipulations were accomplished for the causal connections investigated. No Positive Manipulations or Non-Interventions were reported in the paper, and Proxy convergence was shown only for one of the two hypotheses. (*See* Fig. 9.1.)

To fill out the sort of checklist represented in Table 8.1, one would have to thoroughly search through the entire paper, to make sure that no experiments were omitted from the analysis and that all

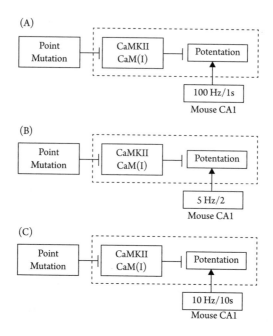

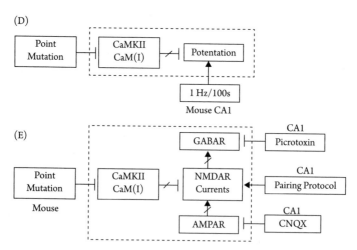

Figure 9.1. Continued

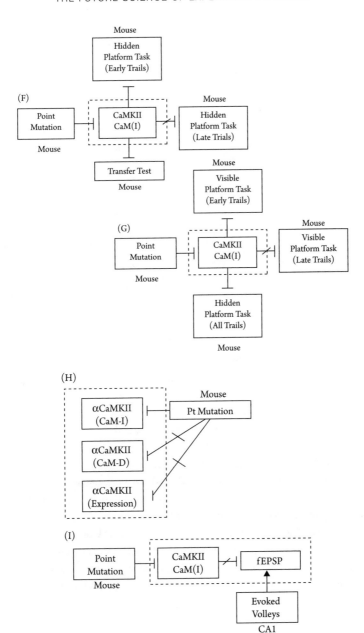

Figure 9.1. Continued

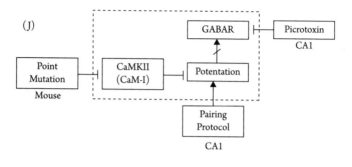

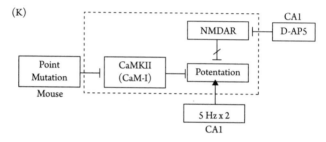

Figure 9.1 Experiment Map for Giese et al. (1998), a paper that was discussed in Chapter 6. The natural system of phenomena is represented inside the dotted line boxes, and manipulations are represented outside of those boxes. The experimental context involves manipulations of CA1 in mice. Negative effects have flat-headed arrows, whereas facilitating effects have pointy arrowheads. When there is no effect, we use broken arrows to represent the experimental finding. αCaMKII can be in a CaM-dependent (CaM-D) or CaM independent (CaM-I) state. αCaMKII (CaM-I) refers to the activated (autophosphorylated) CaMKII state we discussed in earlier chapters. GABAR refers to activity in inhibitory GABA receptors. Picrotoxin is a drug that blocks GABA receptors and CNQX is a drug that blocks AMPA receptors, a kind of glutamate receptor involved in LTP expression. D-AP5 is a drug that blocks NMDA receptors. "Pairing Protocol" refers to a type of LTP-inducing stimulation delivered to both pre- and postsynaptic cells simultaneously. This protocol will stimulate NMDARs, but the normal Target Increase effect was reduced in αCaMKII mutants.

experiments were represented accurately. Some protocol would be needed to ensure the objectivity and systematicity of such an analysis. Such a protocol could reasonably demand that each reported experiment be documented in a manner sufficient to fit causal graphs to each reported experiment in the entire paper. We illustrate the set of causal graphs for the experiments reported in Giese et al. (1998) in Table 9.1.

We've included this complete inventory of the experiments reported in Giese's paper to give the uninitiated a sense of the number of experiments that can be found in a single three-page primary report. Because the number of experiments reported in a single paper can be quite large, it will be important to store each analysis in a well-designed database. If there are any errors or omissions in the analysis, they could then be corrected by revising the database entry. The paper's authors could be contacted with their paper's annotations to help ensure that the representation is accurate.

Table 9.1 Checklist of Convergent Three and Integration Components Accomplished in Giese et al. (1998).

CA1 Mouse	Negative Manipulations	Positive Manipulations	Non-Interventions
CaMKII→LTP	✓		
CaMKII→S. Learning		✓	

Investigating two hypothesized causal connections; *see* our discussion of some of these experiments and results in Chapter 6, section 4.

Once documentation of the sort recommended has been performed for all of the papers in the selected sample, the next logical step would be to start searching for patterns predictive of higher relative citation numbers. For example, as of April 2013, Giese's paper had received 448 citations (ISI Web of Knowledge, queried 04/26/13).. We could compare this number of citations to other papers published in the same year that are retrievable with the search string, "LTP Memory." Those other papers could also be evaluated in terms of the extent that they conformed to the Convergent 3.

One intuitively plausible hypothesis is that—once we control for the novelty of experiments—the extent to which a paper satisfies a Convergent 3 Analysis is positively correlated with the number of citations the paper receives. Note that this prediction does not mean that a comparison between any two papers would follow this rule. Rather, the hypothesis predicts that if enough papers were analyzed, one would see a correlation between the extent to which the different kinds of Connection Experiment are applied and the number of citations a paper receives.

The hypothesis is somewhat simplistic. There may not be many papers reporting more than one kind of Connection Experiment involving the same causal hypothesis. Still, if the results were consistent with the hypothesis, then we would have more reasons to believe that citation measures could be an indicator (if crude) of the information conveyed by a research paper. If the hypothesis failed to hold up, then we could look for other patterns in the data—for example, whether a chain of papers that together satisfy the Convergent 3 Heuristic net higher relative citation.

It would be no surprise if the novelty of a paper dominated predictions of citation. Using the same database, and the Integration approaches discussed, we could operationalize many kinds of novelty. For example, when prevailing evidence for a hypothesis is solely based on one of the legs of the Convergent 3 (e.g., Negative Manipulations), do the first set of experiments using other legs of the Convergent 3 (e.g., Positive Manipulations and Non-Interventions) attract high citation numbers? Multiple hypotheses could be addressed using a single database and could inform through *testing* how, if at all, citation is an indicator of research quality.

5. SIMULATING ALTERNATIVE HISTORIES OF NEUROSCIENCE

Aside from using a map of experiments to integrate, interpret and plan research, we could also use it to ask questions about the impact of prior experiments on current knowledge in neuroscience. If a NEXpath (i.e., a causal network of phenomena) were derived from a database of experiments, then we could investigate the effect that deleting a particular experiment series would have on the connectivity of that network. The changes brought about in a NEXpath by the deletion could serve as an alternative mechanism for evaluating research quality.

For some experiment series, deletions might show very little change, because those experiments yielded little causal information. Looking at experiments from highly informative papers, a deletion from the database might produce a sizeable change in the associated NEXpath, because sometimes a single series of experiments published in a single paper justifies the arrangement of and experimental evidence for several causal connections (recall the Multi-Connection Experiments discussed in Chapter 7). With a metric for the transformations effected in a NEXpath, we could evaluate contributions to knowledge not just in terms of interpersonal influence (e.g., citation) but in terms of logical consequences for a large-scale causal model.

By deleting and adding experiments to our database and observing the changes in the associated NEXpath, we could test hypotheses not only about the contributions made by experiments to knowledge in a field, we could also test the contributions of individual research units. For example, we might delete all of a particular experimenter's work (and perhaps also work directly connected to it) from the database and observe the impact on the shape of the associated NEXpath. We could test the contributions of labs, collaborative research teams, departments, funding agencies, or journals themselves.

The range of research applications for maps of experimental research is in many respects quite astonishing. But one point cannot be overstressed. To run any of these tests, we will need to actually do the work: collect the publications, perform the Integration analyses, build the NEXpaths, and test the measures. This will be no small task.

6. SCIENCE WITHOUT ILLUSIONS

Science is in no small part a quest to shed illusions, illusions whose influence we can only detect through systematic testing. With a framework for cataloging the different forms of experimental practice, and all of the innovations in information technology now within our grasp, we possess the means to turn scientific methods onto the practice of science itself. The molecular and cellular cognition Framework and associated Integration principles described in this book are our first steps toward shedding any illusions that block progress in science. With the knowledge of how research choices are made and how performance in science is rewarded, we seek to develop an empirical science of experiment planning. Scientists' creative potential will not be eclipsed, but it will also not be squandered. We believe that with the clarity of research maps, and with objective tools to evaluate research plans, scientific creativity could finally reach its full potential. With the tools we described here, what has been learned would not be lost and the knowledge that could be gained would not be forfeited. The future is upon us and that future can be engineered to make scientific revolutionaries of us all.

NOTES

Chapter 2

1. We claim no originality for this distinction, and our new terms for these three types of experiments are meant to both offset potentially misleading philosophical connotations pertaining to more familiar terms and to be descriptively accurate.

Chapter 4

1. The way we represent these manipulations is always relative to some description of the agent phenomenon. For example, the NMDA receptor-AP5 experiments described in the previous chapter can be described as a decrease in the probability that NMDA receptors will be activated. Consistency of description is critical in applying the Positive/Negative Manipulation distinction effectively.
2. We say this under the assumption that there is no redundancy in the causes of a phenomenon.
3. This description of syntide2 is an oversimplification. For a more precise description, *see* Hashimoto and Soderling (1987).

Chapter 6

1. *See* Crabbe, Wahlsten, and Dudek (1999) for an example of undependable connections discovered across three separate labs during replication experiments in

behavioral genetics. Small differences in lab conditions led to significant differences in the phenotypes of mice with the same genetic modifications and the same pedigree (i.e., genetic background).

Chapter 7

1. Actually some conventions will minimally require, in addition, the use of U variables to represent all of the independent unmeasured variables that might affect each of the experimental variables we have already mentioned.

Chapter 8

1. Control experiments were used to ensure that CREB-enhanced rats didn't freeze more because of higher anxiety or greater sensitivity to painful stimuli (such as an electric shock).

REFERENCES

Abel, T., P. V. Nguyen, et al. (1997). "Genetic demonstration of a role for PKA in the late phase of LTP and in hippocampus-based long-term memory." *Cell* **88**: 615–626.

Abraham, W. C., B. Logan, et al. (2002). "Induction and experience-dependent consolidation of stable long-term potentiation lasting months in the hippocampus." *The Journal of Neuroscience:* **22**(21): 9626–9634.

Babcock, a. M., D. Standing, et al. (2005). "In vivo inhibition of hippocampal Ca2+/calmodulin-dependent protein kinase II by RNA interference." *Molecular Therapy: the Journal of the American Society of Gene Therapy* **11**: 899–905.

Bach, M. E., R. D. Hawkins, et al. (1995). "Impairment of spatial but not contextual memory in CaMKII mutant mice with a selective loss of hippocampal LTP in the range of q frequency." *Cell* **81**: 905–915.

Barria, A., D. Muller, et al. (1997). "Regulatory phosphorylation of AMPA-type glutamate receptors by CaM-KII during long-term potentiation." *Science* **276**: 2042–2045.

Baudry, M. and Lynch, G. (1981). "Characterizattion of two [^{3}H]Glutamate binding sites in rat hippocampal membranes." *Jounral of Neurochemistry* **36**: 811–820.

Baudry, M., Arst, D., et al. (1981). "Development of glutamate binding sites and their regulation by calcium in rat hippocampus." *Brain Research* **227**: 37–48.

Baudry, M., O. M, et al. (1980). "Increase in glutamate receptors following repetitive electrical stimulation in hippocampal slices." *Life Sciences* **27**(4): 325–330.

Bishop, A. C., J. A. Ubersax, et al. (2000). "A chemical switch for inhibitor-sensitive alleles of any protein kinase." *Nature* **407**(6802): 395–401.

Bliss, T. V. and T. Lømo. (1973). "Long-lasting potentiation of synaptic transmission in the dentate area of the anaesthetized rabbit following stimulation of the perforant path." *J Physiol* **232**(2): 331–356.

Bourtchuladze, R., B. Frenguelli, et al. (1994). "Deficient long-term memory in mice with a targeted mutation of the cAMP-responsive element-binding protein." *Cell* **79**: 59–68.

Buonomano, D. (2011). *Brain bugs: how the brain's flaws shape our lives.* New York, W. W. Norton & Co.

Cain, D. P., D. Saucier, et al. (1996). "Detailed behavioral analysis of water maze acquisition under APV or CNQX: contribution of sensorimotor disturbances to drug-induced acquisition deficits." *Behavioral Neuroscience* **110**: 86–102.

Capecchi, M. (1989). "Altering the genome by homologous recombination." *Science* **244**: 1288–1292.

Cho, J., R. Bhatt, et al. (2012). "alpha-calcium calmodulin kinase II modulates the temporal structure of hippocampal bursting patterns." *PloS One* **7**(2): e31649.

Collingridge, G. L., S. J. Kehl, et al. (1983). "Excitatory amino acids in synaptic transmission in the Schaffer collateral-commissural pathway of the rat hippocampus." *The Journal of Physiology* **334**: 33–46.

Cooke, S. F., J. Wu, et al. (2006). "Autophosphorylation of alphaCaMKII is not a general requirement for NMDA receptor-dependent LTP in the adult mouse." *The Journal of Physiology* **574**: 805–818.

Crabbe, J. C., D. Wahlsten, et al. (1999). "Genetics of mouse behavior: interactions with laboratory environment." *Science* **284**: 1670–1672.

Dash, P. K., B. Hochner, et al. (1990). "Injection of the cAMP-responsive element into the nucleus of Aplysia sensory neurons blocks long-term facilitation." *Nature* **345**: 718–721.

Davis, S., S. P. Butcher, et al. (1992). "The NMDA receptor antagonist D-2-amino-5-phosphonopentanoate (D-AP5) impairs spatial learning and LTP *in vivo* at intracerebral concentrations comparable to those that block LTP *in vitro*." *J. Neurosci.* **12**(1): 21–34.

Dong, Y., T. Green, et al. (2006). "CREB modulates excitability of nucleus accumbens neurons." *Nature Neuroscience* **9**: 475–477.

Egger, G., G. Liang, et al. (2004). "Epigenetics in human disease and prospects for epigenetic therapy." *Nature* **429**(6990): 457–463.

Flexner, J. B., L. B. Flexner, et al. (1963). "Memory in mice as affected by intracerebral puromycin." *Science* **141**: 57–59.

Frankland, P. W. and B. Bontempi. (2005). "The organization of recent and remote memories." *Nature Reviews Neuroscience* **6**: 119–130.

Frey, B. S. and K. Rost. (2008). "Do rankings reflect research quality? Do rankings reflect research quality?" *Research in Economics.* **Zurich:** 1–37.

Gécz, J. (2010) "Glutamate receptors and learning and memory." *Nature Genetics* **42**: 925–926.

Giese, K. P., N. B. Fedorov, et al. (1998). "Autophosphorylation at Thr286 of the alpha calcium-calmodulin kinase II in LTP and learning." *Science* **279**: 870–873.

Grant, S. G., T. J. O'Dell, et al. (1992). "Impaired long-term potentiation, spatial learning, and hippocampal development in fyn mutant mice." *Science* **258**(5090): 1903–1910.

Grant, S. G., M. C. Marshall, et al. (2005). "Synapse proteomics of multiprotein complexes: en route from genes to nervous system diseases." *Human molecular genetics* **14** Spec No. 2: R225–234.

Guzowski, J. F., McNaughton, B. L., et al. (1999). "Environment-speciic expression of the immediate early gene Arc in hippocampal neuronal ensembles." *Nature Neuroscience* **2**(12): 1120–1124.

Han, J. H., S. A. Kushner, et al. (2007). "Neuronal competition and selection during memory formation." *Science* **316**(5823): 457–460.

Han, J.-H., S. a. Kushner, et al. (2009). "Selective erasure of a fear memory." *Science* **323**: 1492–1496.

Hashimoto, Y. and T. R. Soderling. (1987). "Calcium. calmodulin-dependent protein kinase II and calcium phospholipid-dependent protein kinase activities in rat tissues assayed with a synthetic peptide." *Archives of Biochemistry and Biophysics* **252**: 418–425.

Hebb, D. O. (1949). *The organization of behavior; a neuropsychological theory.* New York, Wiley.

Hoffman, D. A., R. Sprengel, et al. (2002). "Molecular dissection of hippocampal theta-burst pairing potentiation." *Proc Natl Acad Sci U S A* **99**(11): 7740–7745.

Josselyn, S. a., C. Shi, et al. (2001). "Long-term memory is facilitated by cAMP response element-binding protein overexpression in the amygdala." *Journal of Neuroscience* **21**: 2404–2412.

Kennedy, M. B., M. K. Bennett, et al. (1983). "Biochemical and immunochemical evidence that the "major postsynaptic density protein" is a subunit of a calmodulin-dependent protein kinase." *Proceedings of the National Academy of Sciences of the United States of America* **80**: 7357–7361.

Lee, Y.-S. and A. J. Silva. (2009). "The molecular and cellular biology of enhanced cognition." *Nature Reviews Neuroscience* **10**: 126–140.

Lisman, J., H. Schulman, et al. (2002). "The molecular basis of CaMKII function in synaptic and behavioural memory." *Nature Reviews Neuroscience* **3**: 175–190.

Lisman, J. E. (1985). "A mechanism for memory storage insensitive to molecular turnover: A bistable autophosophorylation kinase." *Proceedings of the National Academy of Sciences* **82**: 3055–3057.

Lisman, J. E. and M. A. Goldring. (1988). "Feasibility of long-term storage of graded information by the Ca2+/calmodulin-dependent protein kinase molecules of the postsynaptic density." *Proc Natl Acad Sci U S A* **85**: 5320–5324.

Levenson, J. M. and J. D. Sweatt. (2005). "Epigenetic mechanisms in memory formation." *Nat Rev Neurosci* **6**(2): 108–118.

Lledo, P. M., G. O. Hjelmstad, et al. (1995). "Calcium/calmodulin-dependent kinase II and long-term potentiation enhance synaptic transmission by the same mechanism." *Proc Natl Acad Sci U S A* **92**(24): 11175–11179.

Lømo, T. (1966). "Frequency potentiation of excitatory synaptic activity in the dentate area of the hippocampal formation." *Acta Physioligica Scandanavica* **68**(Supplement 227): 128.

Lømo, T. (2003). "The discovery of long-term potentiation." *Philosophical transactions of the Royal Society of London. Series B, Biological sciences* **358**: 617–620.

Mansuy, I. M. and S. Shenolikar. (2006). "Protein serine/threonine phosphatases in neuronal plasticity and disorders of learning and memory." *Trends in Neurosciences* **29**: 679–686.

Marr, D. C. (1971). "Simple memory: a theory for archicortex." *Phiosophical Tranactions of the Royal Societty London* **262**: 23–81.

Martin, S. J., P. D. Grimwood, et al. (2000). "Synaptic plasticity and memory: an evaluation of the hypothesis." *Annual Review of Neuroscience* **23**: 649–711.

Martin, S. J. and R. G. Morris. (2002). "New life in an old idea: the synaptic plasticity and memory hypothesis revisited." *Hippocampus* **12**(5): 609–636.

Matynia, A., S.A. Kushner, and A.J. Silva. (2002). "Genetic approaches to molecular and cellular cognition: a focus on LTP and learning and memory." *Annu Rev Genet* **36**: p. 687–720. PMID: 12429705.

Mayford, M., J. Wang, et al. (1995). "CaMKII regulates the frequency-response function of hippocampal synapses for the production of both LTD and LTP." *Cell* **81**(6): 891–904.

Mayford, M., M. E. Bach, et al. (1996). "Control of Memory Formation Through Regulated Expression of a CaMKII Transgene." *Science* **274**: 1678–1683.

McHugh, T. J., M. W. Jones, et al. (2007). "Dentate gyrus NMDA receptors mediate rapid pattern separation in the hippocampal network." *Science* **317**: 94–99.

Migaud, M., P. Charlesworth, et al. (1998). "Enhanced long-term potentiation and impaired learning in mice with mutant postsynaptic density-95 protein." *Nature* **396**(6710): 433–439.

Milner, B. (1965). "Visually-guided maze learning in man: Effects of bilateral hippocampal, bilateral frontal, and unilateral cerebral lesions." *Neuropsychologia* **3**: 317–338.

Miller, S. G. and M. B. Kennedy. (1986). "Regulation of brain type II Ca2+/calmodulin-dependent protein kinase by autophosphorylation: a Ca2+-triggered molecular switch." *Cell* **44**(6): 861–870.

Morris, G. M. (1981). "Spatial localization does not require the presence of local cues." *Learning and Motivation* **260**: 239–260.

Morris, R. G. M., E. Anderson, et al. (1986). "Selective impairment of learning and blockade of long-term potentiation by an N-methyl-D-aspartate receptor antagonist, AP5." *Nature* **319**: 774–776.

Morris, R. G. M. (1989). "Synaptic plasticity and learning: selective impairment of learning in rats and blockade of long-term potentiation in vivo by the N-methyl-D-aspartate receptor antagonist AP5." *J. Neuroscience.* **9**(Sept.): 3040–3057.

Morris, R. G. and M. B. Kennedy. (1992). "The Pierian Spring." *Current Biology: CB* **2**(10): 511–514.

Moser, E. I., M. B. Moser, et al. (1994). "Potentiation of dentate synapses initiated by exploratory learning in rats: dissociation from brain temperature, motor activity, and arousal." *Learning & Memory* **1**(1): 55–73.

Neves, G., S. F. Cooke, et al. (2008). "Synaptic plasticity, memory and the hippocampus: a neural network approach to causality." *Nature Reviews Neuroscience* **9**: 65–75.

Paulsen, O. and E. I. Moser. (1998). "A model of hippocampal memory encoding and retrieval: GABAergic control of synaptic plasticity." *Trends Neurosci* **21**(7): 273–278.

Pearl, J. (2000). *Causality: models, reasoning, and inference.* Cambridge, U.K.; New York, Cambridge University Press.

Posner, M. I. and G. J. DiGirolamo. (2000). "Cognitive neuroscience: origins and promise." *Psychological Bulletin* **126**(6): 873–889.

Poulsen, D. J., D. Standing, et al. (2007). "Overexpression of hippocampal Ca 2 + / calmodulin-dependent protein kinase II improves spatial memory." *Journal of Neuroscience Research* **739**: 735–739.

Russ, T. a., C. Ramakrishnan, et al. (2011). "Knowledge engineering tools for reasoning with scientific observations and interpretations: a neural connectivity use case." *BMC Bioinformatics* **12**: 351.

Sah, P., R. F. Westbrook, et al. (2008). "Fear conditioning and long-term potentiation in the amygdala: what really is the connection?" *Ann N Y Acad Sci* **1129**: 88–95.

Sanderson, K. (2011). "Curation generation." *Nature* **470**: 295–296.

Saucier, D. and D. P. Cain. (1995). "Spatial learning without NMDA receptor-dependent long-term potentiation." *Nature* **378**(6553): 186–189.

Scoville, W. B., and B. Milner. (1957). "Loss of recent memory after bilateral hippocampal lesions." *Journal Of Neurology, Neurosurgery, and Psychiatry* **20**: 11–21.

Silva, A. J., C. F. Stevens, et al. (1992a). "Deficient hippocampal long-term potentiation in o-calcium-calmodulin kinase mutant mice." *Science* **257**: 201–206.

Silva, A. J., R. Paylor, et al. (1992b). "Impaired spatial learning in l-calcium-calmodulin kinase mutant mice." *Science* **257**: 206–211.

Silva, A. J., Y. Zhou, et al. (2009). "Molecular and cellular approaches to memory allocation in neural circuits." *Science* **326**(5951): 391–395.

Simkin, M. V. and V. P. Roychowdhury. (2005). "Stochastic modeling of citation slips." *Scientometrics* **62**: 367–384.

Simkin, M. V. and V. P. Roychowdhury. (2007). "A mathematical theory of citing." *Journal of the American Society for Information Science* **58**: 1661–1673.

Slutsky, I., N. Abumaria, et al. (2010). "Enhancement of learning and memory by elevating brain magnesium." *Neuron* **65**(2): 165–177.

Spirtes, P., C. Glymor, and R. Scheines. (2000). *Causation, Prediction, and Search* (2nd ed.). Cambrige, MA: MIT Press.

Tan, E. M., Y. Yamaguchi, et al. (2006). "Selective and quickly reversible inactivation of mammalian neurons in vivo using the Drosophila allatostatin receptor." *Neuron* **51**(2): 157–170.

Tan, S. E. and K. C. Liang. (1996). "Spatial learning alters hippocampal calcium/calmodulin-dependent protein kinase II activity in rats." *Brain Research* **711**: 234–240.

Tillman, R. E., D. Danks, et al. (2009). *Integrating locally learned causal structures with overlapping variables*. Advances in Neural Information Processing Systems 21, Proceedings of the Twenty-Second Annual Conference on Neural Information Processing Systems, Vancouver, British Columbia, Canada, December 8–11, 2008, MIT Press.

Treves, A. and E. T. Rolls. (1994). "Computational analysis of the role of the hippocampus in memory." *Hippocampus* **4**: 374–391.

Wang, H., E. Shimizu, et al. (2003). "Inducible protein knockout reveals temporal requirement of CaMKII reactivation for memory consolidation in the brain." *Proceedings of the National Academy of Sciences of the United States of America* **100**: 4287–4292.

Wayman, G. A., Y. S. Lee, et al. (2008). "Calmodulin-kinases: modulators of neuronal development and plasticity." *Neuron* **59**(6): 914–931.

Wiltgen, B. J., G. A. Royle, E. E. Gray, A. Abdipranoto, N. Thangthaeng, N. Jacobs, F. Saab, S. Tonegawa, S. F. Heinemann, T. J. O'Dell, M. S. Fanselow, and B. Vissel, *A role for calcium-permeable AMPA receptors in synaptic plasticity and learning*. PloS one, 2010. **5**(9).

Yin, J. C., J. S. Wallach, et al. (1994). "Induction of a dominant negative CREB transgene specifically blocks long-term memory in Drosophila." *Cell* **79**: 49–58.

Zamanillo, D., R. Sprengel, et al. (1999). "Importance of AMPA receptors for hippocampal synaptic plasticity but not for spatial learning." *Science* **284**: 1805–1811.

Zhou, Y., J. Won, et al. (2009). "CREB regulates excitability and the allocation of memory to subsets of neurons in the amygdala." *Nature Neuroscience* **12**: 1438–1443.

INDEX